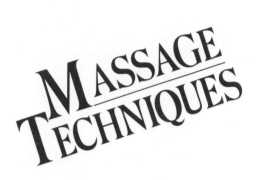

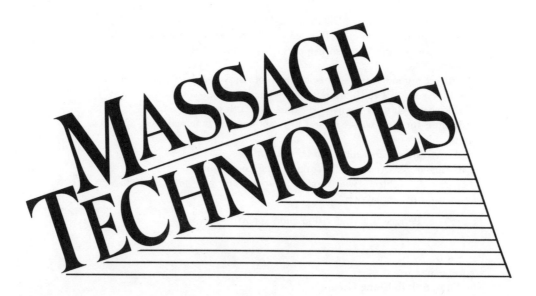

MASSAGE TECHNIQUES

D. Baloti Lawrence

A PERIGEE BOOK

In writing this book it has been my good fortune to be surrounded by the best in human character. The quality of those persons involved has not only touched me but also helped to shape the quality and tone of this work.

To direct a good play requires the help of many people who remain behind the scenes. I did not do it alone! Thank you to:

Dr. Richard Hansen for his dedication to health care.

Adrienne Ingrum, whose insight has captured the practicality of my visions.

Sue Christmas, who would not let me stop.

Mr. Eugene Lawrence II for support when needed most.

My darling children, who seemed to understand why most of 1985 was spent at my typewriter.

Thank you, Perigee, for your vision and support.

Perigee Books
are published by
The Putnam Publishing Group
200 Madison Avenue
New York, NY 10016

Ebet Roberts—Photography
Frederick Bush—Illustrations
Special Contributions—Carolyn Nelson, Towan Lawrence,
Frank Algarin, Ina Vistica, Elinor Bowles, Roberta Roll,
Habbiba Mathew, Nuri Bird, Barry Brown, Judea Lawton,
Deborah Tobias, and William Flocco

Library of Congress Cataloging-in-Publication Data

Lawrence, D. Baloti.
    Massage techniques.

    Includes index.
        1. Massage—Therapeutic use.   2. Massage.
I. Title.
RM721.L39   1986   615.8′22   85-21454
ISBN 0-399-51189-X

Printed in the United States of America
            6   7   8   9   10

*This book is dedicated to the support of all our
efforts to obtain success and happiness through the expression
of physical, emotional, and social well-being . . .*

—D. BALOTI LAWRENCE

CONTENTS

INTRODUCTION TO MASSAGE 9

1 ■ SPORTS MASSAGE 16

2 ■ SHIATSU AND ACUPRESSURE 31

3 ■ SWEDISH MASSAGE 49

4 ■ REFLEXOLOGY/FOOT MASSAGE 70

5 ■ MYOTHERAPY (or Bonnie Prudden Technique) 92

6 ■ THE ALEXANDER TECHNIQUE 102

7 ■ HYDROTHERAPY 118

8 ■ ESTHETIC MASSAGE 128

RESOURCES 155

INDEX 157

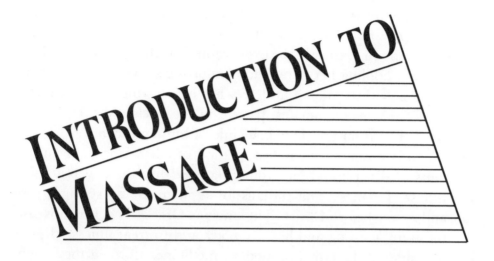

INTRODUCTION TO MASSAGE

This book will provide you with a variety of available massage techniques both for therapeutic and relaxation purposes. It will enable you, in many instances, to help yourself or others, using simple techniques, or it will direct you to the proper bodywork professional. As you become aware of an energizing or relaxation technique or learn methods to alleviate a headache or a sore throat or prevent a sports injury, my hope is that you will be more in control of your body, mind, and spirit.

These days many people who seek help from physicians have complaints of psychosomatic illnesses that are caused by tension and anxiety coupled with an inability to cope with daily stress. This is especially true for people who live in big cities.

Once you realize the reason for certain physical problems, you can change your reaction to stress-producing situations and begin to eliminate the problem. Your brain is the master of your body, and when you select your reactions and emotions rather than let them rule you, you have acted as your own best doctor. Negative feelings eventually find their way to your body in the form of some physical imbalance.

While it is wise to avoid negative emotions, it is not healthy to keep feelings pent up without expressing them in some form, because of this mind and body connection. Massage and bodywork can help.

While the definition of *massage* is specifically the kneading, manipulation, or application of methodical pressure and friction to the body, the term *bodywork* is used to include the more general application of touch. Perhaps you've heard the expression, Touching is healing. Think of a mother cuddling her baby and comforting him with a gentle and soothing touch. Imagine an athlete who, just having won a game, is carried aloft by his teammates, patted on the back and even hugged. Massage is based on the same principle of human touch.

Massage is probably the oldest method of alleviating pain and the symptoms of disease and for promoting good health. It was used by the Chinese, Japanese, and Indians for suppleness and strength three thousand years before Christ. The ancient Greeks and Romans used it to maintain a strong and healthy body and to treat illness. Hippocrates, considered the father of modern medicine, affirmed the benefits of massage and the need for its skilled use by physicians.

Although for a few decades massage fell into disrepute, it is once again gaining recognition as an invaluable therapeutic tool that can be used in both the prevention and the treatment of illness and injuries. The skilled application of touch has many benefits, from the treatment of damaged muscles to the revitalization of such crucial organs as the heart and lungs.

Massage can be used to maintain and enhance the health and well-being of the entire body. All the body's major systems—skeletal, muscular, circulatory, nervous, respiratory, digestive, and urinary—can be positively affected by massage and body manipulation. Massage benefits each system of the body in specific ways.

Skeletal System

- Correct posture and body balance are maintained.
- Muscular tension, which eventually causes structural problems, is reduced.

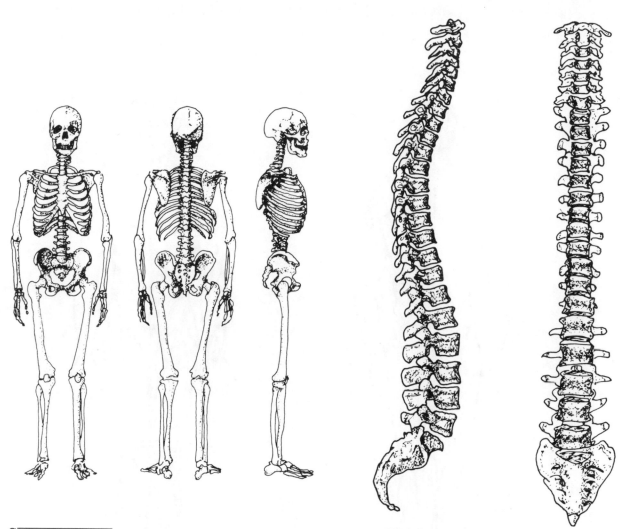

Skeletal system (l to r): front view, back view, side view. *Spine front view and side view.*

- The flow of nutrients to the bones is increased.
- The elimination of waste matter is promoted.

Muscular System

- Muscle tension is relieved and spasms are relaxed.
- The supply of blood and nutrients to muscles is increased.

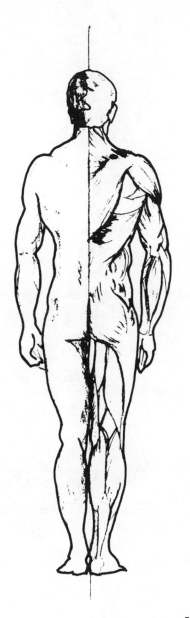
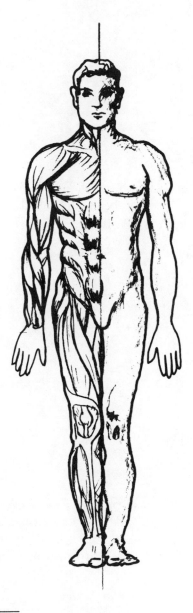

Muscular system.

- Waste matter from muscles (especially lactic acid) is eliminated.
- Tone is restored to flaccid muscles, partially compensating for lack of exercise and inactivity because of illness or injury.
- Muscle adhesions resulting from injury are eliminated or prevented.
- Flexibility and strength of joints is increased.

Circulatory System

- Blood circulation is improved.
- The supply of oxygen and nutrients to cells throughout the body is increased.
- Strain on the heart is eased through the normal return of blood to this vital organ, especially in cases of forced inactivity due to illness or injury.
- Lymph is moved efficiently throughout the body, strengthening the immune system and eliminating toxic waste.

Nervous System

- The nervous system can be either sedated or stimulated, depending on the technique used.
- The nervous system can be balanced, thereby affecting all the systems of the body.

Respiratory System

- Breathing patterns are improved.
- Long-term respiratory difficulties such as asthma and bronchitis are relieved.

Digestive System

- Waste products are pushed out of the system, maintaining regularity and relieving constipation.
- Spastic colon is relieved.

Urinary System

- The kidneys are massaged, thereby cleansing the blood and toning the entire system.
- Swelling is reduced due to the elimination of fluids.

Because of these benefits, it may serve you well to pamper your body with massage. However, if you are experiencing cardiovascular, heart, or severe respiratory problems, it may be wise to consult your physician before utilizing the techniques presented in this book.

The use of skilled touch through massage is good not only for your physical condition but also for your emotional well-being. Psychologists and other behavioral scientists have long recognized the necessity of touch for full personal development. It has been suggested that many psychological disorders experienced by human beings are caused by lack of physical contact.

The image of the masseur or masseuse who taps, kneads, rubs, and pounds our bodies to make them feel better is only partially accurate. Other systems exist that do not use these techniques. There is a world beyond Swedish massage or even sensual massage!

In this book I will outline several different types of massage or bodywork systems, which are based on different physical principles. Some of the systems are structure based and stem from Western traditions of science and medicine. These systems view the body in terms of its structural components—muscles, bones, tissues, organs. Other systems (for example, acupressure and Chua Ká) are energy based and stem from the Eastern belief that all living matter possesses a life-giving energy or vital force that circulates throughout the organism and must be kept strong and free flowing to maintain health. In Japanese philosophy, this energy is called *ki;* in yoga, it is called *prana.* A third group of bodywork systems is based on the idea of electrochemical and neuromuscular reflexes that can be stimulated within the body. These systems include Polarity, Rolfing, and Osteopathy.

The bodywork systems described in this book are merely a few of the most popular types that are practiced around the world. They were selected because most of the systems can be used for self-care as well as administered by another person. It will be up to you to decide whether to do the techniques on yourself, learn to do them with a partner, or hire a professional practitioner. Other systems not mentioned in this text include: Amma, Chua Ká, Trager, Hellerwork, Chiropractic, Rechian Therapy, Applied Kinesiology, Do In, Feldenkrais, Naprapathy, and Rolfing.

While each of the systems affects the body in a slightly different way, all the systems have one thing in common: when properly applied, they will definitely make you feel better. More than this, they can help you change your life and get more out of every day. They will increase your energy level, stimulate mental alertness, and aid in total relaxation.

The popularity of total approach to fitness is growing—an approach that considers the mental as well as the physical well-being of people. Many think that traditional medical science may need reexamination. Others believe that traditional medicine is the only way. However, reports on nutrition, exercise, and stress management conclude that the best of both worlds would be optimal.

High achievers must expend large amounts of time and energy. Whatever your life-style is—whether you're an athlete whose livelihood depends on a clear mind and a healthy body, an executive who must be mentally alert and physically fit to face a hectic schedule, or a homemaker and mother whose schedule has its own intense demands— physical and mental well-being is important. While massage is not a panacea, it is an important component of a healthy and vital life-style. So get to know ways of preventing and relieving your basic aches and pains. This will give you a greater sense of freedom and activity. Taking time to pamper yourself will help preserve your natural youthfulness and help create a more beautiful, vibrant you!

Use your common sense, consult your physician, check out the qualifications of your bodywork practitioner, then enjoy, enjoy, enjoy!!!

ONE
SPORTS MASSAGE

■ What Is Sports Massage?

This growing field of bodywork is a method of alleviating pain and bringing relief to tired or aching body parts. It is particularly useful in relieving or reducing the possibility of cramps and muscle spasms in dancers and athletes.

■ Benefits of Sports Massage

Sports massage stimulates the glands, nerves, blood vessels, muscles, and connective tissues. It helps empty the blood and lymph vessels and bring fresh fluid into these areas, thereby eliminating poisons and waste matter from the tissues and improving circulation. Specifically, it can be helpful with:

- relaxation
- elimination of stiffness and temporary paralysis

16

- reduction of swelling
- tissue regeneration
- increased range of motion and freedom in movement
- increased circulation to an injured body part
- loosening tight or contracted muscles
- firming weak muscles

While the benefits of sports massage far outweigh the possible adverse effects, massage should be avoided when an area is bruised, cut, or harbors a torn ligament or fracture, or where there is infection. It should also be avoided in any situation for which deep manipulation is contraindicated.

■ Background and History of Sports Massage

With the growing concern about physical fitness, more and more people are engaging in athletics or other forms of strenuous exercise. Because of added stress to the body and poor exercise habits, many of these new sports buffs are experiencing injuries and strains. While massage has always been used in such sports as boxing and football, professional as well as amateur athletes are increasingly using massage both to prevent and to treat injuries.

One of the leading exponents of sports massage is Marquetta K. Hungerford, Ph.D., who has taught and practiced massage therapy throughout the country. Dr. Hungerford combines massage therapy, physical therapy, and nutrition in the treatment of athletes. She is past director of education of the American Massage Therapy Association and is the founder of the American Massage Therapy Institute, Costa Mesa, California.

■ Basic Principles and Philosophy of Sports Massage

Although massage is used to treat sports injuries, it is perhaps even more important as a preventive measure. It has been clearly demonstrated that massage helps bring about increased physical endurance, greater relaxation, and stronger muscles. When these conditions are present, injury is less likely to occur. Massage also helps create the balance and efficient movement that promotes speed, power, and endurance. These attributes help the athlete perform at peak level without endangering the body.

There is a fine line between physical conditioning and physical breakdown or injury. Emotional or personality factors or stress and tension may also contribute to lower resistance in the body. When the body is in this state of low resistance or when muscle parts are weakened, injury is likely to occur.

Therefore, in planning any exercise or athletic regimen, remember that your body has its limits, which are governed by your individual physical makeup and endurance, level of skill, emotional state, and preparation.

Sports massage today has a greater and more efficient meaning for the athlete, not just as a relaxing rubdown but as a method of increasing performance skills. Because the body is a system of integrated functions, all systems working together—it is important they do just that—harmoniously work together. When this occurs, all systems are go!

■ Sports Massage Techniques

Many different massage techniques are beneficial in preparing the body for strenuous activities and/or treating injuries that can result from such activities. Two of the most valuable techniques are *muscle kneading* and *range of motion*.

Muscle Kneading

Muscle kneading is routinely used by dancers and athletes during warmups. It can be applied easily anywhere on the body except the shins, bony joints, and skull.

Kneading, which is experienced by the body as an alternation between relaxation and compression, consists of two steps:

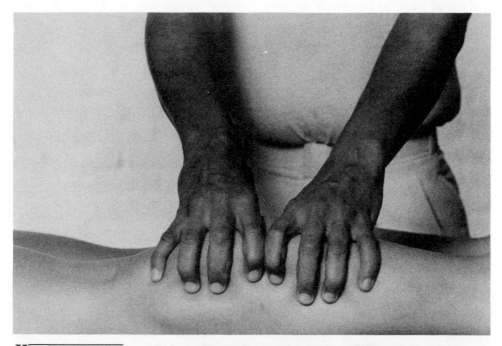

Hand position for muscle kneading. After applying a small film of oil on the area to be worked on, grasp the muscle with a squeezing action of your hand. If the muscle is properly oiled, it will immediately begin to slip out of your hand. As the muscle slips from your hand, quickly grasp it with your other hand. The muscle will continue to slide from hand to hand as it is pressed, creating a rolling effect. Continue the kneading for about thirty seconds to one minute on most areas, but for about five minutes on the back. Here buttocks are kneaded, an especially useful technique for swimmers and dancers.

1. After applying a small film of oil to the area to be worked on, grasp the muscle with a squeezing action. If the muscle is properly oiled, it will immediately begin to slip out of your hand.

2. As the muscle slips from your hand, quickly grasp it with your other hand. The muscle will continue to slide from hand to hand as it is pressed, creating a rolling effect. Continue the kneading for about thirty seconds to one minute on most areas, but for about five minutes on the back.

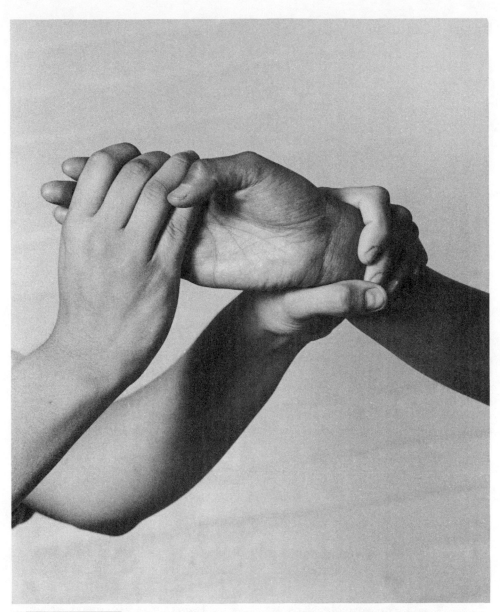

*R*ange of motion applied to hands and wrists. When muscles are not used, they weaken and deteriorate. Often joint injuries result in pain and limited movement. Range-of-motion exercises increase movement and activate muscles. Using both hands, one holding wrist, the other grasping fingers, rotate on the axis of wrist joint 5 times in each direction. This is an especially useful technique for players of all racquet sports.

Range of Motion

Range of motion is a gentle movement for evaluating the condition of the joints, increasing their flexibility, and eliminating tightness and tension.

Each joint has a normal range of motion. The condition of the muscles associated with each joint can be evaluated by taking it through its normal range.

1. To improve the condition of the joints and associated muscles, slowly try to rotate the joint through its normal range of motion, moving it in all ways possible. Hold the body part to be worked on in your hand to give it support as you move the joint. Slowly rotate the joint six times in one direction and then six times in the opposite direction. Repeat the cycle three times.

2. Repeat gentle range of motion exercises periodically—about every two or three hours—until the tightness or limitation of movement is lessened.

Massage can be used to treat many types of sports injuries, such as:

- sciatica
- muscle tears
- tennis elbow
- bursitis
- frozen shoulder
- knee pain
- backaches
- headaches
- neck sprains
- finger sprains

Each individual's body is different. Individual stamina and weaknesses as well as the condition of the body and emotions have a great deal to do with the types of injuries likely to be incurred by participation in sports. Nevertheless, certain sports are particularly hazardous for specific body parts. The following is a list of the most popular sports and the body parts that are most likely to be affected:

SPORT	BODY PART AFFECTED
TENNIS	elbow, arms, wrist, ankles
GOLF	back, feet, neck, shoulders
SWIMMING	back, eyes, legs, skin
BASKETBALL	shoulders, head, knees, ankles
RACQUETBALL	head, back, wrists, fingers, legs
WRESTLING	back, arms, legs
BOXING	head, stomach, eyes
WEIGHT LIFTING	arms, back, legs
JOGGING	feet, ankles, legs, chest
SKIING	legs, ankles, arms, skin
AEROBIC DANCE	legs, ankles, back, stomach, arms

The following is a general list of the types of sports injuries likely to be incurred:

- general aches and pains
- muscle tears, pulls, sprains, stiffness, cramps
- bursitis—inflammation
- strains
- cuts, punctures
- bruises
- friction burns
- dehydration
- frostbite
- fractures

■ Sports Massage to Relieve or Prevent Injuries

In addition to massage, other techniques can be valuable for preventing serious injury to the body, such as taping, use of protective gear, and exercise.

Taping provides support to ligaments and joints and maintains joint alignment. It includes the following steps:

1. Shave hair from the area to be taped.
2. Use gauze as an underlining to protect the area from irritation.
3. Use good-quality tape that is strong yet flexible.
4. Wrap the tape firmly but not so tightly that circulation will be inhibited.

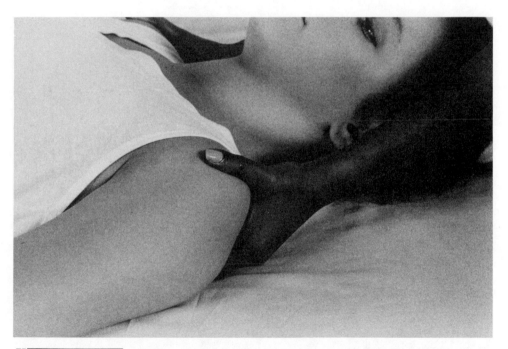

Kneading the stiff shoulder. First knead with fingers, moving across shoulder from neck. Then press down on shoulders. Place hands on top of shoulders and lean in, applying gentle pressure. It is important to tone these muscles and skin attached to facial structures. Constricted shoulder or neck muscles may cause tension or even wrinkles in facial structures as their attachment makes one affect the other.

Support pads should be used on knees and shoulders to cushion the area from abuse. The eyes should be protected with goggles, and helmets should be worn to reduce injury to the head in sports in which those areas are in jeopardy.

Stretching exercises, which warm up the muscles and increase their flexibility, are vital for anyone participating in a strenuous activity. Like massage, they strengthen the connective tissues by stimulating the flow of oxygen and nutrients.

A good fitness program for sports participants should include massage, hydrotherapy, exercise, proper nutrition, relaxation techniques, and protective measures such as taping and proper sports gear.

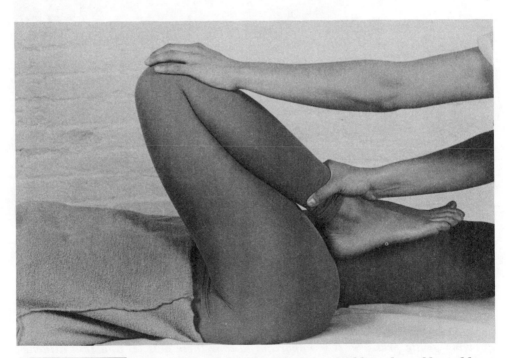

Knee exercise and leg stretch to prevent knee injuries. Holding the ankle and knee, lean into knee, and gently stretch.

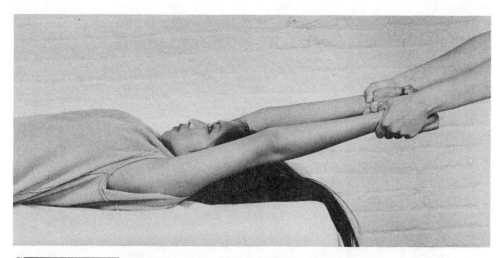

Shoulder and neck cramps may be prevented and relieved by this pleasant stretch. Grasp the wrists and lean back while pulling the arms slightly. Hold for approximately thirty seconds and release. Repeat 3 times.

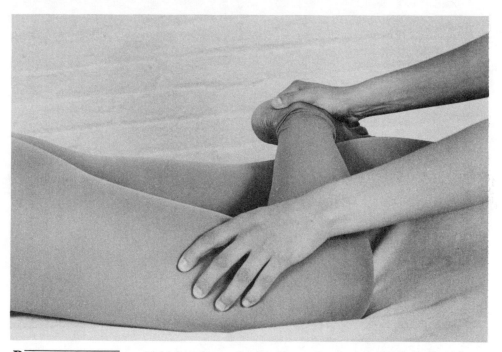

Relieving leg cramps. Fold leg across back of knee. Begin just below buttocks and apply firm pressure, finishing with the toes.

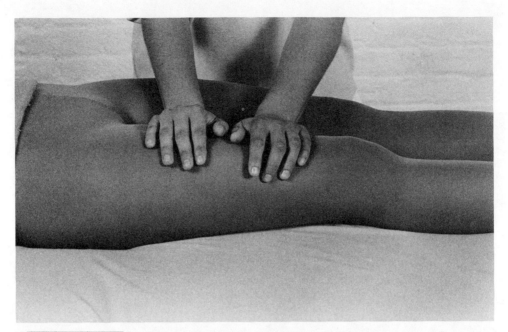

Sports massage to prevent muscle tears in legs. Apply firm pressure to leg, using palm of hand. Then rock the muscle. Free your hands before beginning by shaking them rapidly for approximately thirty seconds.

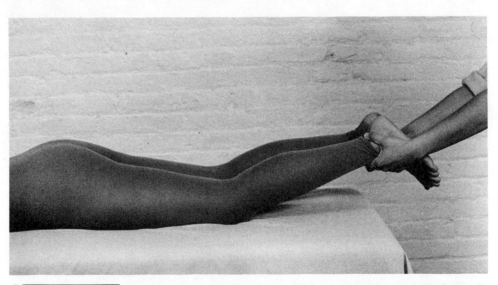

Leg stretch relieves tight and tense leg muscles. Grasp the ankles with both hands; lean back and pull. Let your weight balance you as you lean.

26   MASSAGE TECHNIQUES

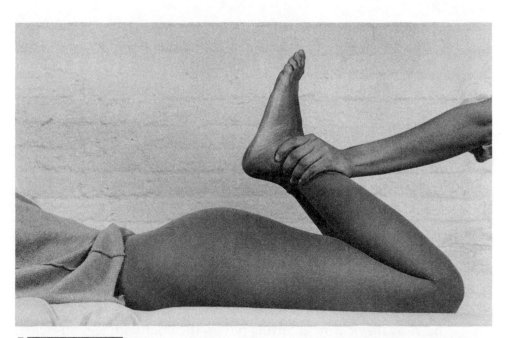

Lower back and knee stretch to prevent and relieve lower back injuries. Lower back pain is often the result of tight thigh muscles. This movement stretches both the back and the lower legs.

■ Self-exercises for Strengthening Muscles

Quick, forceful movements may lead to back pains. Muscles should be strong yet flexible. Good posture is also important. It is also important to maintain proper tone in the abdominal muscles, as they offer valuable support to the lower back.

1. *Sit-ups.* Lie on your back with your knees bent. Curl your body up toward your knees, keeping your buttocks flat on the floor.
2. *V-sit.* Lie flat on your back. Lift the upper torso and the legs at the same time.
3. *Leg lift.* Lie flat on your back with hands behind the neck

and legs extended with feet together. Raise both feet, keeping knees straight, about ten inches from floor. Hold for approximately ten seconds. Repeat three times.

4. For flexibility in the lower back, stand up straight, feet together. Reach down as far as you can. Do not bend the knees. Try touching the floor. Once you reach your maximum stretch, inhale deeply, exhale and stretch a bit further.

5. Hold a weight (20–40 lbs.) over your head with arms extended. Lower it behind your head, bending your elbows. Repeat six times.

   For strengthening hands and wrists, squeeze a rubber ball twenty-five times with each hand. Repeat exercise as often as possible.

   For strengthening legs, lean against a wall and stand on your toes. Hold for 10 seconds, then return to heels.

6. *Body stretch exercise.* Sitting flat on the floor with legs stretched out in front of you, reach for your toes until you feel the stretch in the back of your leg. Remain still for ten seconds, relax, and then repeat. Remember to inhale and exhale freely.

■ Self-Massage for Athletes

Done before an athletic activity, sports massage increases the flexibility of muscles, allowing for freer movement. Included as part of a warmup, it also gives the body a sense of well-being and confidence.

If the activity places heavy stress on a particular body part, a massage of those areas will prevent tension and pain. Self-massage provides the opportunity to limber these areas in a warmup routine. There are several basic techniques you can apply to yourself, shown here.

After an athletic activity, sports massage can be applied to relax and relieve the tension built up during the activity. In addition, warming and caring for muscles directly after a strenuous activity provides the body with a sense of relaxing pleasure after the high adrenaline of athletic activity.

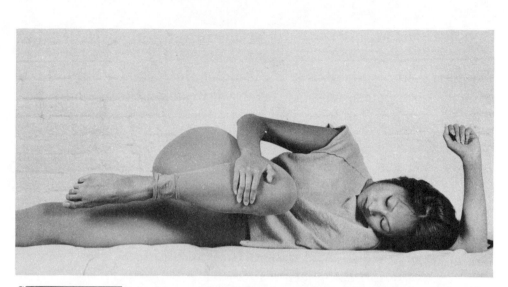

S̲e̲l̲f̲-massage for tight legs, especially the front of the legs. This should be done before running, swimming, or skiing, to release tension and tightness.

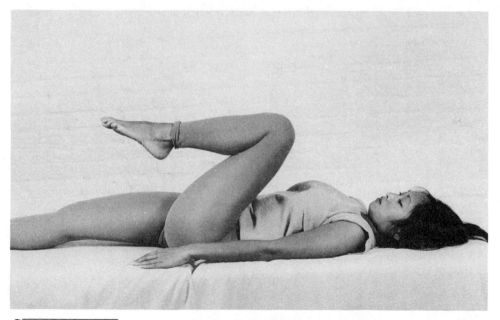

S̲e̲l̲f̲-massage to strengthen stomach muscles. Hold leg at a 45-degree angle, inhale, and count to ten. Release slowly, then repeat.

■ Training and Certification

Sports massage therapists are increasing in number. Their backgrounds may include physical therapy, general massage therapy, athletic instruction and training, nursing or other sports specialties. Because sports and fitness participation is increasing rapidly by the general public, the need to prevent and care for injuries is also increasing. This means the field is wide open for sports massage therapists. For information on training and certification contact:

> Dr. Marquetta K. Hungerford, Ph.D.
> American Massage Therapy Institute
> 204 E. Sixteenth Place #1
> Costa Mesa, CA 92627

■ Locating a Sports Massage Practitioner

Contact Dr. Hungerford at the address just given.

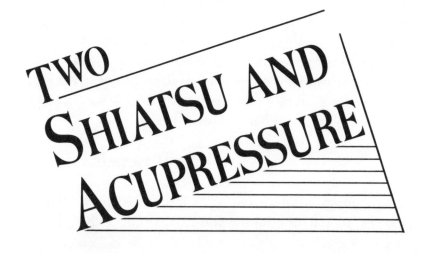

TWO
SHIATSU AND ACUPRESSURE

■ What Is Shiatsu?

Shiatsu is a system of Japanese bodywork that uses gentle manipulation combined with finger and hand pressure on the body's energy meridians. By releasing blocked energy, shiatsu relieves pain and tension, corrects the functioning of the internal organs, and treats specific conditions of illness. It follows the same principles as the Chinese healing method of acupuncture, but where acupuncture uses needles, shiatsu and acupressure use finger pressure. Acupressure has, in fact, often been called acupuncture without needles.

Acupressure and shiatsu are often mentioned together. Their philosophies both outline an Oriental perspective on healing. Acupressure stimulates pressure points that exist throughout the body by manipulating the body's energy where tension accumulates and where it blocks the free flow of energy.

The original approach to acupressure by practitioners was based entirely on an instinctive knowledge of where to touch. Eventually certain places of the body became known as points of relief.

Shiatsu and acupressure differ in that shiatsu may include certain body manipulations and movements, while acupressure, like acupuncture, rests solely on the stimulation of energy meridians.

Shiatsu is used at its best as a preventive measure through which the individual is made more aware of internal and external imbalances that can lead to discomfort and illness. If illness does occur, this sensitivity allows early detection and treatment. In this way, each person can take responsibility for his or her own health.

■ Benefits of Shiatsu

The overall objective of shiatsu is to establish the body's normal physical and emotional functioning and to bring the body into harmony with its environment.

The following are some of the specific benefits that can be obtained through shiatsu:

- Aches, pains, and fatigue are relieved, as well as such conditions as dizziness and insomnia.
- Internal complaints ranging from kidney and bladder problems to indigestion, breathing difficulties, and liver complaints can be affected. As the energy in the meridians is balanced, the corresponding body systems are brought into normal functioning, improving circulation and hormonal activity.
- Mental and emotional discomfort is also affected. As the body's energy is balanced, stress is reduced and the person feels calmer and more relaxed. He or she gains more mental clarity and relates to other people in a more harmonious way. A sense of emotional balance is achieved that allows the person to use emotions as a full and productive part of living.
- Diet and life-style changes often occur naturally as a result of regular shiatsu sessions.

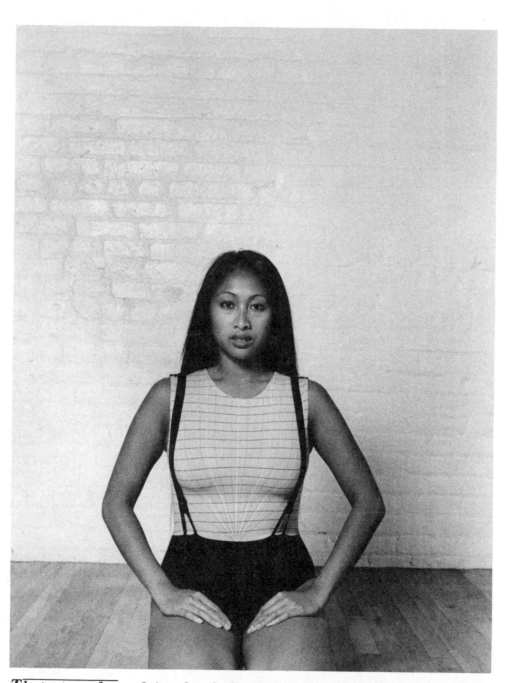

The purpose of many Oriental methods of bodywork is to create harmony and well-being in the body. Shown: Oriental position for meditation and relaxation.

While shiatsu is excellent for providing quick relief from certain problems, it is most effective when administered regularly over time, since the treatments have a cumulative effect, especially on deeper constitutional deficiencies.

■ The History of Shiatsu

Shiatsu, which originated in Japan, has been recognized worldwide for about seventy years. The word means "finger" (*shi*) and "pressure" (*atsu*).

The system is based on Chinese medical theories that were introduced to Japan about a thousand years ago. At that time, *amma*, a form of massage similar to Western techniques, was well known and used extensively by Japanese physicians, who were required to learn it in order to understand the body's structure and the body's meridian lines, or energy pathways. Eventually *amma* came to be used only for simple problems such as back pain and neck tension. Often practiced by blind people, it gradually became associated with pleasure and relaxation.

When the Japanese government issued regulations requiring that *amma* practitioners be licensed, many changed the name of their work. They integrated techniques from *do-in* (a yoga-based system of self-massage) and *amma* and then added their personal touch. Shiatsu was the name given to this bodywork system. As *amma* became used more for pleasure, shiatsu became a very technical form of medical treatment, eventually borrowing from Western medical theory to explain its results.

In the past, there were many different schools of shiatsu in Japan. Three of the most well known were those of Tokujiro Namikoshi, Katsusuke Serizawa, and Shizuto Masunaga. Today there are different approaches to the system: the classic, rather brusque style; the more popular softer approach; the barefoot style; and many offshoots. In the United States, Wataru Ohashi has developed *Ohashiatsu*, which has done much to bring shiatsu to the attention of the general population.

■ Basic Principles and Philosophy of Shiatsu

Shiatsu is based on an approach to health that differs considerably from the usual Western view. The Eastern philosophy of health emphasizes the body's own healing powers rather than the use of drugs or surgery to cure physical problems.

Shiatsu is used to discover the cause of illness or discomfort and to treat the problem at its origin. The practitioner helps restore the normal functioning of the individual's organs and systems so that the illness is fought by the body's own mechanisms. Consequently, in shiatsu the client may actually feel worse temporarily before getting better. Western medicine, on the other hand, tends to focus on the relief of external symptoms and the control of pain. Also, a shiatsu client is helped to become aware of imbalances in the body and to take responsibility for preventing illness as well as for restoring and maintaining a healthy balance. As a result, the client is expected to become less dependent on health care practitioners.

According to the theory on which shiatsu is based, meridians, or pathways of energy, flow throughout the body and govern the body's life force, which in turn feeds the body's organs. While the existence of these meridians is not proved in Western medicine, the sensitive person can feel rushes of energy within the body that are like warm, surging sensations along the meridians. It is also possible to feel *tsubos*, which are small indentations under the skin, along the meridians. These 361 *tsubos* correspond to different internal organs. About 90 are used in shiatsu practice.

According to Eastern medical theory, seventy-two meridians exist at different layers in the body. Traditional shiatsu uses the twelve meridians closest to the surface of the body. Six are in the arms and six are in the legs. Each governs a different organ in the body, and they are paired according to their function. For example, the kidney meridian is paired with the bladder meridian. Their functions complement each other, since both are concerned with detoxification, purification, and hormonal secretions. Two additional meridians used in shiatsu are on a level slightly deeper than the other twelve. The *governing vessel* and the *conception vessel* are concerned with the functioning of the *ki,* or life energy flow, and run up the center of the back and the center of the front of the body respectively.

When a person is healthy, the energy flows freely throughout the body, along the meridians. When illness or pain occurs, the energy is trapped. Most of us have experienced this in a mild form when we feel a painful sensation on our skin or get a muscle cramp.

Energy may become blocked for a variety of reasons: poor posture, poor eating habits, lack of exercise, injury, stress, or emotional upset. If a blocked condition persists, it may affect the internal organs severely and manifest itself as a serious illness, such as kidney stones, liver or heart problems, diabetes, or even cancer. When the energy is kept flowing and the internal organs are functioning properly, the individual lives in a state of balance and health.

The foundation of shiatsu lies in Eastern thought and philosophy, which view the individual as a microcosm of the universe. One of the major underlying concepts of Eastern thinking is the principle of *yin/ yang,* or the duality of energy in the universe. Yin embodies the feminine; quiet, passive, cool, downward, dark, and inward aspects. Yang is masculine; active, bright, outward, warm, and upward. Everything in the universe contains both these qualities, although one may be more dominant in general or at a particular point in the life cycle.

Eastern philosophy also views nature and life as a cyclical flow of energy throughout the universe. Everything that exists consists of five basic elements: fire, metal, earth, water, and wood. Each element influences and creates another. Thus, wood is used to produce fires. Fire creates earth by making ashes. Earth, over time, turns into metal ore. Water nourishes the earth and gives life to plants and trees, which create wood. Each element also has specific characteristics and is associated with a particular color, season, time of day, flavor, sound, smell, food, emotion, part of the body, and many other aspects of life.

In turn, each meridian is associated with one of the five elements.

MERIDIAN PAIRS		ELEMENT
YIN	YANG	
Heart	Small intestine	Fire
Heart constrictor	Triple Heater	Fire*
Stomach	Spleen	Earth
Lungs	Large Intestine	Metal
Kidney	Bladder	Water
Liver	Gall bladder	Wood

This cyclical concept suggests that energy never stops or dies—it is simply transformed. Similarly, if one meridian is blocked and lacks energy, another will have excess energy. In order to affect the meridian that is actually causing the problem, a practitioner may work to free the energy in another meridian.

Diagnosis is an integral part of the practice of shiatsu. Practitioners may work on a particular meridian in order to bring about quick superficial relief from symptoms such as pain, dizziness, and nausea. In order to bring about significant changes, however, the practitioner must understand thoroughly the underlying cause of the imbalance. This is done through various diagnostic techniques that are used together to achieve a full picture of what is going on internally and externally.

Do-shin means "through observation," which includes looking at the shape of the face, the color and texture of the skin, the nails, the hair, posture, and many other external aspects.

Bun-shin means "sound." The practitioner will listen to the tone of the voice, for sounds of breathing and digestion, and sounds in the joints or other parts of the body.

*These two meridians are supplemental fire. The heart constrictor governs circulation and sex, and the triple heater governs the temperature in the body.

Mon-shin involves questioning the individual about how he or she feels and thinks.

Setsu-shin is diagnosis through touch. This includes pulse diagnosis, in which the condition of the six pairs of meridians is felt through the separate and corresponding pulses in the wrist. Another part of setsu-shin is *ampuku*, or *hara* diagnosis. In Eastern teaching, the *hara* is the energy source and the seat of the soul. It is located in the abdominal region and is bounded by the pubic bone, the crests of the hipbones, and the inner edge of the rib cage up to where the two sides of the rib cage meet. All energy comes in, is transformed, and leaves through the *hara*, which is the meeting point for yin/yang. All meridians have their source of energy here, and there are points for each major organ.

It is believed that all disease stems from the *hara;* hence, the practitioner can detect imbalances through touching the hara and can begin to release energy blockages during this process.

Diagnosis through *setsu-shin* is always treatment as well. As the practitioner touches and palpates the area, energy is released and dispersed. The practitioner will usually go to the *hara* first in diagnosing and then later to verify diagnosis and assess the results of treatment. It must be remembered that diagnosis in shiatsu does not mean looking for a disease. Rather, it is to assess the individual's condition and to improve that person's life.

When a practitioner uses *setsu-shin,* he or she is diagnosing the condition of the *hara*, meridians, and *tsubos*. As the various points are touched and lightly pressed, the practitioner feels that the point is either *kyo* or *jitsu*. These are Japanese words with meanings similar to the Chinese terms of yin and yang. A *kyo* point will feel soft, flaccid, weak, lacking in energy, and perhaps cool. *Jitsu* points feel stiff, hard, excessive in energy, and perhaps warm. The *kyo* point draws one into the body; the *jitsu* point resists the touch.

A *jitsu* condition is one in which energy has been blocked, built up, and stagnated. However, it is usually temporary, the overall constitution of the individual being strong, and it releases relatively easily with simple stimulation. The process of normalizing the *jitsu* area is known as *sedation,* although *dispersal* might give a more accurate description of what actually happens.

The *kyo* condition, characterized by depleted energy, is more difficult to treat and indicates chronic stagnation and weakness. A *kyo* condition exists behind every serious illness. Deep holding pressure is required to balance and tone this condition. Sometimes a point may feel *jitsu* initially, but as the practitioner maintains pressure, the point reveals its true *kyo* nature.

As the meridians are touched, usually a particular pair will be more *kyo* or *jitsu* than the others, and within that pair, one will be more *kyo* and the other more *jitsu.* The *kyo* points are generally more important to locate than the *jitsu,* as they indicate a deeper imbalance. Therefore, the practitioner will usually start by balancing the *kyo* points to build up the depleted energy. This draws some of the energy away from the *jitsu* areas and normalizes them. The practitioner may or may not need to further balance the *jitsu* areas later. However, since there are no hard and fast rules in shiatsu, the practitioner may, if the person is a particularly *jitsu* or yang type, start with balancing the *jitsu* areas first and the *kyo* areas afterward.

Part of shiatsu diagnosis also involves the emotions and feelings that the client is experiencing. Psychological states correlate to each meridian, and these states vary according to whether a *kyo* or a *jitsu* condition exists. For example, a person with a *kyo* condition in the kidney meridian may experience anxiety, fear, lack of determination and desire, and pessimism. A *jitsu* condition may produce feelings of impatience, "workaholic" tendencies, restlessness, complaining, and nervousness. Consequently, psychological characteristics help the practitioner determine the client's condition, where the energy is trapped, and how to proceed with treatment.

The simultaneous nature of diagnosis and treatment gives shiatsu its uniqueness. Both modalities occur together throughout the session, and no two sessions are alike, even for the same complaint. A person has a slightly different internal condition each time, and the session depends on that individual, not on a set order and style of treatment.

Two complementary techniques are used in shiatsu: gentle stretching with range of motion manipulations (rotating a body part at its joint to the fullest extent possible) and pressure.

Gentle stretching and range of motion manipulations are usually performed at the beginning of the session. They help warm up the body by stimulating circulation and stretching the meridians. This brings the meridians to the surface of the body and makes them more accessible to the practitioner.

The practitioner applies pressure to parts of the body by using his or her fingertips, palms, thumbs, elbows, or sometimes even feet and toes. It is always applied in a vertical downward direction. The basic techniques for applying pressure are palming and thumbing. Palming is particularly good for stretching and adjusting body parts and for relieving *jitsu* conditions. It is performed with the entire hand relaxed and resting on the body. One or both palms can be used. When both hands are used, one is placed on top of the other. Palming may be done in a slightly undulating, circular, rubbing, or grasping motion, or with simple downward pressure. *Kenbiki* is a palming technique that uses the hand in a pushing and pulling motion to warm up an area by drawing the blood to it.

Generally, the practitioner should not apply pressure in a sudden or jerky manner. If resistance is felt, he or she must move slowly, gradually increasing the pressure so that there will not be excessive pain. Some discomfort may be felt by the client during or after the session and perhaps even two or three days afterward. This is caused by trapped, stagnant energy and will diminish as the body's energy is balanced.

In order to keep the energy flowing, the practitioner should synchronize his or her breathing with that of the client and should maintain physical contact with the client's body. The practitioner must work from his or her own *hara* in order to use the body's weight correctly. The *hara* is the body's center of gravity and is located in the pelvic area. The practitioner's *hara* should be close to the client's body and over the area being worked on. In his way, the practitioner's weight, not the force of the hands or arms, is used to control the pressure. By working from the *hara,* the practitioner achieves a sense of oneness with the client. The practitioner's body becomes aware and the hands become receptive and sensitive, which enables them to "see" the blocked energy and help redirect it.

A shiatsu session is conducted on the floor with the client lying on a mat or carpet. The floor supports the body against the downward pressure exerted by the practitioner. Loose, comfortable clothing is worn by both client and practitioner. A tranquil, softly lit environment is desirable for maximum relaxation and receptivity.

In shiatsu, the client/practitioner relationship is extremely important. The client must be willing to acknowledge what is happening to him or her physically and emotionally and must be ready to participate in the process. Effective shiatsu is promoted by patience and commitment, trust and openness between the two people.

■ Training, Certification, and Careers

There is no licensing specifically for shiatsu. Any licensing that is required is dictated by a particular state's licensing laws concerning massage.

Certification in shiatsu can be obtained in many ways: through state accredited schools, various health education organizations, and training programs taught by individuals. Certification varies and can take anywhere from a few months to over a year. However, like most bodywork systems, extensive experience is required to become a skilled practitioner. To practice shiatsu in its true form requires in-depth knowledge of Eastern medical theory, which can take years. On the other hand, the basic skills needed to give beneficial *shiatsu* for mild complaints and minor imbalances can be mastered in a relatively short time.

Information about schools and certification programs can be ob-

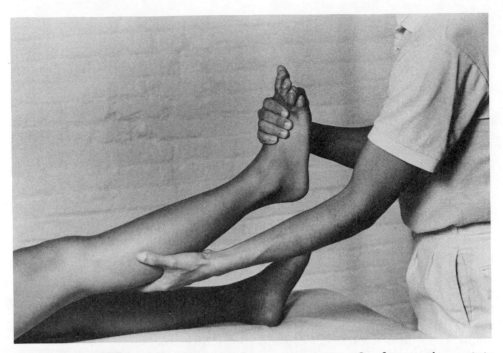

Leg rotation stimulates bladder and kidney energy centers. One leg at a time, rotate the entire leg in circles, releasing tension at the hip area.

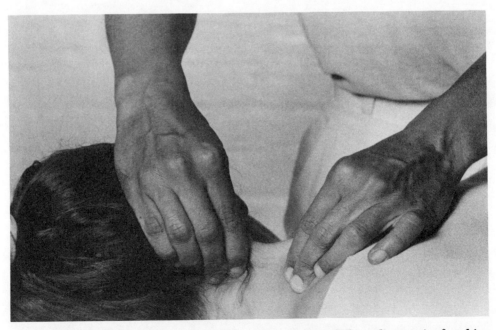

A gentle stretch on the neck, moving from top to bottom, helps relieve a tired, aching back. Gently apply finger pressure for ten seconds. Repeat 3 times. Then apply pressure with both thumbs. Use the pad of the thumb and gently lean in, adding pressure.

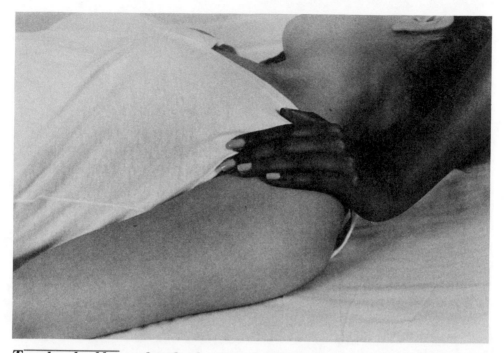

To relax shoulders and neck, place your hands on top of each shoulder and apply gentle pressure toward chest. Then rock shoulders side to side.

tained through the American Massage Therapy Association, the Alliance for Massage Therapists, and the Shiatsu Education Center of America.

■ How to Locate a Practitioner

While there is no central organization of shiatsu practitioners, they are found in all parts of the world and throughout the United States. The greatest concentrations are on the East and West coasts. To locate a practitioner in your locality, contact a state accredited school that teaches shiatsu or a holistic health center in your area.

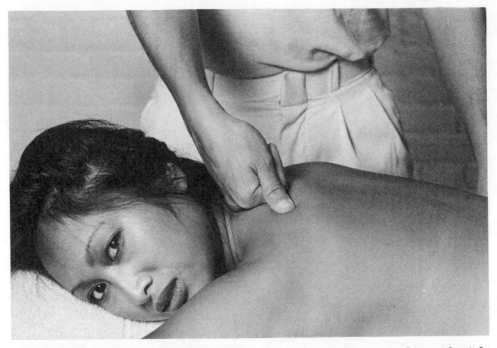

Pressure point for neck and upper back. It is approximately one inch outside right corner of left shoulder blade. Press down and in, and hold for about ten seconds.

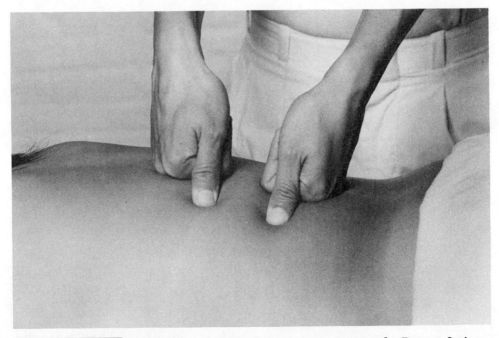

Pressure points for back pain. Press in for seven to ten seconds. Repeat 3 times. Do this to both sides of back.

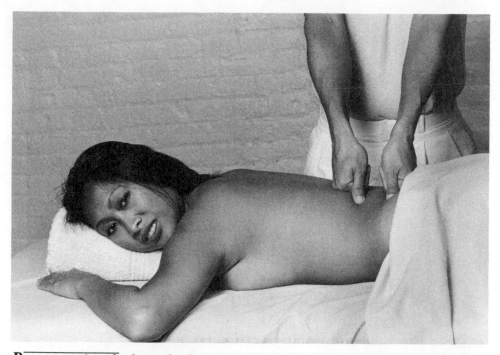

Pressure points for lower back. Press in gently for seven to ten seconds. Repeat 3 times. Do this on both sides of back.

■ Acupressure

Though similar to shiatsu in many ways, acupressure uses no body manipulation techniques, only pressure to the body's energy meridians. Acupressure is particularly useful in treating back pain—any pain in the back that may be characterized by dull, continuous pain or tenderness in the muscles or any attachment from the muscles, ligaments or tendons, particularly in the lower area of the back (known as the lumbar region or, further below that, the sacroiliac region). Pain is often transferred to the leg from the back. The sciatic nerve may lead to a particular type of pain known as sciatica. Infection or abnormality in another part of the body (particularly some internal disorders) may be a cause of back pain.

Another cause may be a disorder of the vertebrae (the series of ladderlike steps that lead from the spine through the back). If the vertebrae or ladderlike steps are out of line or out of order, they may press down on a vertebral disc, causing pain.

Other disturbances are strain or sprain or structural inadequacies if the spinal column is not supported properly by the ligaments, muscle injury, spasms, or inflammation. There are also certain emotional or psychogenic factors that may lead to back pain.

If the pain in the lower back has existed for some time and is fairly constant and very sharp, it could be the result of a ruptured or disintegrated disc. Poor athletic or dance training, poor posture, and carelessness when lifting objects are also causes of back pain, as lifting objects that are too heavy can place an undue stress or strain on the back area.

Work tables and desks that are too high can cause your shoulders to raise, bringing tightness and pain to the back area. Working or sitting in the same position for extended periods of time and acquiring bad habits of posture can also lead to back pain.

Very often internal disorders, particularly the organs located around the lumbar regions in the lower back, such as the kidneys, liver, or pancreas, can cause pressure or an internal pain reflecting itself in the lower back. Fractures from injuries or dislocations to the vertebrae can also cause lower back pain.

Remember, chronic pain is a pain that occurs over and over and over; acute pain is one that simply has its origin at a given time and goes away, perhaps to reoccur.

Some signs of imbalance in the back are:

1. Neck tilted to one side.
2. Hunched shoulders.
3. Pain in the back.
4. Pain in the chest area.
5. Pain in the abdomen. Also, weak abdominal muscles or muscles that are flaccid may lead to lower back pain. Since the

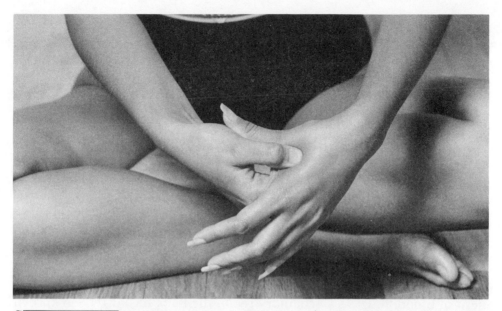

Self-technique for headache. To locate this point, place the first line of the opposite thumb into the web of the open opposite hand at the point just outside the top of the thumb. Gently press 3 times for about seven seconds each.

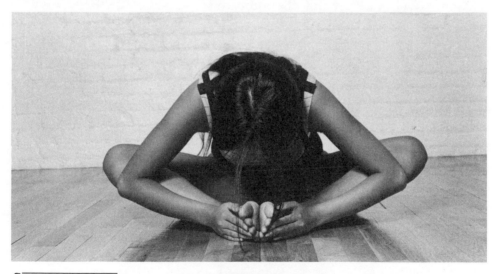

Shiatsu self-technique for back and thigh stretch and toning of organs. With both legs folded and soles of feet touching, grasp each foot and slowly lean toward the floor.

abdominal region or the stomach muscles are the muscles that support the lower back, it is necessary that these muscles be strengthened or strong or the lower back will have a tendency to lean forward, placing undue pressure on it, thus causing lower back pain.

6. Curved spine may also cause imbalances in the back. It may be kyphosis, lordosis, or scoliosis, depending upon where the curvature exists (if it's at the top, middle, or bottom part of the spine). Some of these, particularly scoliosis, have been known to be corrected by exercise, but only by working with a professional who understands the cause of this condition.

Special methods of massage or exercise that help relieve back pain may be geared around the relaxation of tense muscles. The improvement of blood flow to a particular area in the back has also been known to be helpful. Muscle reeducation (placing the muscle in correct position to return it to its normal function and breaking bad habits forced upon the muscular system) may be necessary. In cases of excessive muscle tension, psychotherapy may be indicated.

■ Education and Certification

Certification in acupressure is a procedure that varies from state to state. Local rules and regulations dictate the requirements and responsibilities of the practitioner. In some states, the law requires a state-approved school to administer its own program and offer certification to its students. Other states offer certification after the applicant has passed a state exam. Schools offer programs for beginners or advanced students. Curricula always include an introduction to Oriental health philosophy, the meridian system, techniques, and practical application. Students are encouraged to practice as they learn.

THREE
SWEDISH MASSAGE

■ What Is Swedish Massage?

Swedish massage is a body manipulation system that duplicates the movements of Swedish gymnastics and other types of exercise. Swedish gymnastics includes bending, stretching, flexing, and rotating the muscles and joints. It contains forty-seven positions and over eight hundred movements. In Swedish massage, the practitioner imitates these movements in order to stimulate circulation, increase muscle tone, and create an all-around balance to the structure and function of the muscular-skeletal system.

■ Benefits of Swedish Massage

Massage has been used throughout the ages because it works. The advantages of skillful Swedish massage are evidenced in many ways and include pain relief, relaxation, improved circulation, better nutritional absorption, increased muscle tone, and better mobility in the joints, as well as rehabilitation of muscles and damaged tissues. The mind and spirit can also experience benefits—clarity of thought, relief from mental and emotional tension, and freer expression. Together these benefits make you a more fully functioning, self-confident individual.

Swedish massage also can be used to exercise the muscles passively to maintain stretch, mobility, and tone. This is excellent for people who experience muscle fatigue, weakness, and atrophy resulting from lack of exercise or forced inactivity due to illness, injury, exhaustion, overweight, or aging.

Massage is extremely useful after many kinds of injury or surgery, since it keeps the muscle fibers loose and keeps them from sticking together. It can lessen or prevent the formation of scar tissue. Swelling is reduced as waste products and fluids are carried from the site, thus lessening pain. As excessive swelling resulting from injuries to tendons and ligaments is reduced, pain is lessened, movement is made easier, and rehabilitation and recovery are hastened. As nutrients are allowed to enter the area easily, minerals needed for repair are provided, especially in the case of fractures.

The following are some of the specific benefits of massage:

- *Skin* Clogged pores are opened and dead cells removed, enabling respiration to take place more easily. This helps keep the skin smooth, supple, well nourished, and radiant. Stimulation of the glands beneath the skin, such as the sweat glands, leads to heightened activity, again cleansing the skin and promoting new cell growth. General respiration and absorption of the skin is improved as oxygen is taken in, nutrients are absorbed, and waste products are eliminated.
- *Nerves* Sensibility in the nerve endings is heightened, allowing the person to become either more sensitive to touch or lessening irritability and hypersensitivity, such as to pain or fabrics.
- *Muscles* When muscles become overloaded with toxic waste

products, such as uric and lactic acids, fatigue and eventually pain occur. This reaction is common after injury, overexertion, or the prolonged, intense performance of athletes. Massage will help move these waste products from the tissues, preventing soreness and overfatigue and allowing nutrients to rebuild and strengthen the tissues. Often, if an athlete receives a Swedish massage after a competition, he or she will experience none of the fatigue, soreness, or pain that are commonly felt the following day.

- *Circulation of lymph and blood* Massage increases the return of blood through the veins to the heart, and massage strokes are always done toward the heart for this reason. This allows new blood to be pumped through the arteries and capillaries. It has been shown that the capillaries actually expand, bringing blood to all the tissues of the body. This can be seen when the skin becomes reddened after sustained pressure on the skin.

    Lymphatic fluid is moved through the body by means of gravity and muscular activity. If this activity is heightened through massage, the drainage will be greater.

    Edema is lessened as fluid is moved and brought into circulation. As lymphatic circulation is increased, the body can eliminate toxins and waste products and fight infection more easily and efficiently.

    Better circulation throughout the body leads to better nutritional absorption and functioning because, as the old material is carried out, new fluids and nutrients are allowed to enter at a faster rate. Metabolism and organ function improve, and digestion and elimination proceed more effectively.

- *Blood pressure* Improved circulation can, in some instances, reduce blood pressure, which has been known to drop as much as twenty points after a session. CAUTION: Abdominal massage is the exception, as it raises blood pressure. Except for that, massage is excellent for stress reduction and the hypertensive patient. More hemoglobin and more red and white blood cells are brought into circulation. Anemia may be alleviated through massage, as the blood cells become unstuck from the walls of the blood vessels.

- *Peristalsis* Massage stimulates the action of peristalsis, which moves material through the intestines and finally through the bowels. Excretion of inorganic minerals and salts via the kidneys is facilitated and urine flow is increased, making massage useful in various kidney and bladder ailments. Constipation and diarrhea can be helped, and toxemia resulting from blockages or inflammation of various organs is decreased.

- *Heart and lungs* The heart itself can be stimulated directly by massage, making it an invaluable aid in emergencies such as heart attacks. The lungs can benefit greatly as mucus and secretions are dislodged, dispersed, and eliminated. People with asthma, emphysema, pneumonia, and other respiratory disorders will find positive changes and relief through skilled Swedish massage.

- *Nervous system* Both motor and sensory nerve endings are stimulated through massage. Hypersensitivity of the sensory nerves is decreased and their functioning is improved. The nerves that affect secretions, digestion, and other internal processes can be stimulated, especially through abdominal massage.

- *Self-image* An important benefit of massage is the "sense of self" that it induces. Physically, the sense of the body's boundaries, the different functions of the muscles, and how the body moves contributes to knowledge about oneself and helps remove self-imposed limitations. Once you know how your body moves and functions, you can feel comfortable in exploring all the possibilities. This transfers to the psychological realm also. The physical and psychological effects of massage are, thus, all interrelated and affect one another and the person as a whole being.

Massage can have calming benefits in cases of nervous exhaustion, emotional upset, panic, fear, and anxiety. By helping a person relax, it generates the release of emotional tension and the subsequent ability to deal with stress.

Massage can have a stimulating, a sedative, or even an exhausting effect on the nervous system, depending on the length and type of treatment. Hyperactive children can be calmed and convulsions diminished through the relaxation of the nervous system induced by massage. Some forms of paralysis have been known to respond to massage techniques.

Massage can also be a magnificent way to "get away from it all," to escape from daily pressures and concerns. You might call it a mini-vacation! It has even been used successfully to assist drug and alcohol abusers going through withdrawal, as well as the emotionally disturbed.

■ Background and History of Swedish Massage

Peter Hendrik Ling of Sweden (1776–1839) is credited with developing the system of Swedish massage that exists today. He was a well-educated man who had studied fencing and eventually opened his own fencing school. As a young man, he developed a severe case of arthritis. When no help could be found in Europe, he traveled to China, where he studied massage with Taoist priests and was cured of his arthritis.

He returned to Sweden thrilled with his new knowledge and, based on his study of Oriental techniques and his knowledge of anatomy and physiology, formulated a system of Swedish gymnastics. He established the Royal Institute of Gymnastics in Stockholm in 1814. Here he taught the use of his system for military training and medical purposes. The medical version incorporated active movement, massage, and manipulation to exercise the muscles. The system was widely accepted in Europe and was used by many practitioners and physicians.

Although Ling developed the basis of Swedish massage, his successors did much to expand and refine it. A French system was developed, using soothing manipulations, especially to the head, neck, face, and arms, to promote smooth and youthful skin. The German system incorporated the Swedish approach with the use of different types of hydrotherapy. The English system expanded the techniques into what is now known as physiotherapy. Swedish massage was introduced to the United States during the latter part of the nineteenth century and was used during World Wars I and II to treat the injured and hospitalized.

Massage, as it was used at that time, was actually a form of physiotherapy and incorporated exercise, hydrotherapy, and manipulation. Most massage was practiced in hospitals, where doctors routinely prescribed it for their patients. Gradually, however, the nonmedical massage became increasingly popular. In 1955, laws were passed forbidding anyone without a nursing degree or four years of college from working in a hospital. These two factors contributed to the decline of therapeutic massage, and massage eventually became associated with sensuality.

During the late 1960s and early 1970s, physical therapists and nurses began to rediscover the value of touch and hands-on contact with patients and people in pain and discomfort. Although massage is still often thought of exclusively in terms of its sensual benefits and the medical field does not yet acknowledge its true value, it has gradually regained acceptability as a viable means for promoting health and recovery from many conditions. Health clubs, spas, and the holistic health movement have done much to promote the value of massage for well-being and dispel public fears and negativity.

■ Basic Principles and Philosophy of Swedish Massage

Medical practitioners and behavioral scientists are gradually coming to realize the importance of touch. Studies show that deprivation of touch can lead to emotional disturbance in infants that can affect them into their adult years, causing maladaptive socialization and difficulties in forming relationships.

Sensitive physical contact through the hands creates immediate communication between individuals and has a nurturing and healing effect. The skilled practitioner is able to use this nonverbal communication to determine when changes in technique should be made. Consequently, machines, no matter how well designed, cannot have the healing power of a pair of well-trained and sensitive hands.

Massage is not a panacea and must be used correctly. The effective practice of massage depends on a knowledge of anatomy, physiology, physical and emotional development, and various massage techniques. The condition of the person must be properly assessed so that it can be determined if massage will be beneficial or whether massage is contraindicated. Most people can give an emotionally soothing massage simply by applying a caring touch. However, in order to bring about changes within the body, thorough knowledge and skill are required.

One of the major principles of Swedish massage is that circulation and flexibility are the keys to good health. The body is an integration of many systems—circulatory, lymphatic, respiratory, digestive, endocrine, nervous, muscular, and skeletal. If any of them ceases to work fully, blockage, stagnation, and restriction occur, minimizing activity and producing pain, fatigue, or possibly disease. The proper use of massage can eliminate blockages and increase the circulation of blood and other body fluids, the mobility and range of motion of the joints, and the power and balanced action of the muscles. Massage can help keep the body's various systems in a state of free-flowing health, so that disorders do not develop and the individual's general health improves.

■ Swedish Massage Techniques

Swedish massage consists of five basic strokes: effleurage, petrissage, friction, tapotement, and vibration.

- *Effleurage*, a French word for "stroking," usually begins and ends massage on a particular body part. It also may be interspersed with other strokes. Effleurage is a gliding stroke that is executed by sliding the hands evenly over the body surface with long strokes, always in the direction of the heart, directing energy toward the vital center of life.

The stroke begins lightly and gradually increases in pressure, tapering off at the end. It can be applied with the palms of one or both hands, depending on the size of the body part being massaged. When small surfaces on the body are involved, either the ball of the thumb or the fingertips may be used.

This stroke warms up the tissues in preparation for deeper work and soothes muscles, tissues, and nerves. It can relax, induce sleep, and decrease pain. It increases the rate of blood flow back to the heart, allowing new blood to flow to the tissues and more oxygen and nutrients to be received and utilized. By moving the tissues in an upward direction (toward the heart, neck, and head), it helps the lymphatic fluid flow toward the drainage ducts around the chest and neck area, cleansing the body.

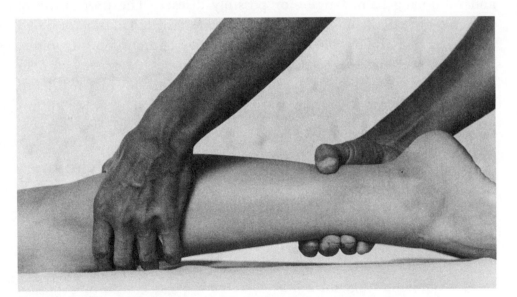

Effleurage: stroking the leg to release leg tension and stimulate muscles.

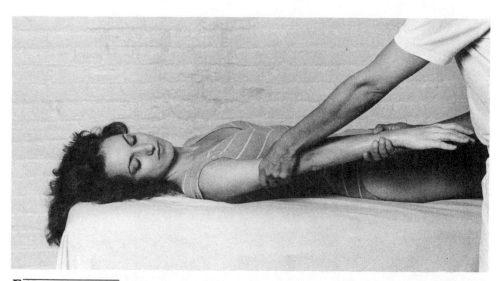

Effleurage: stroking the arm and hands. Begin at shoulders and use long, firm strokes toward fingertips. Tennis and golf players will appreciate the increase of circulation around a stiff elbow.

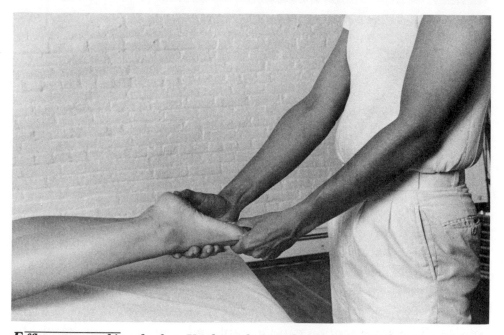

Effleurage: stroking the feet. Use long, firm strokes. Begin at the ankles and stroke toward toes. This helps relieve tired feet, tightness, and tension.

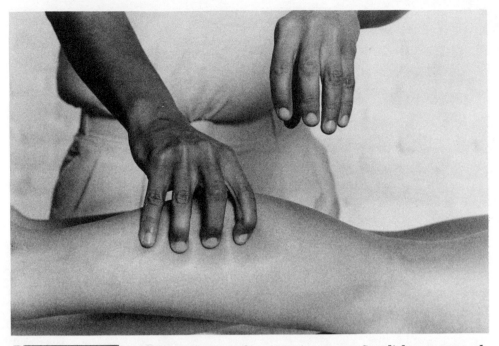

P̲e̲t̲r̲i̲s̲s̲a̲g̲e̲: kneading calf muscle. Kneading is an important Swedish massage technique. Think of kneading dough. Place hands on leg. Fingers should be flat over muscle area. Alternate hands by lifting one, then the other.

■ *Petrissage,* which is a French word for "kneading," is a rhythmic lifting, squeezing, pressing, and rolling stroke that is performed with the hands either stationary or traveling slowly along the length of a muscle or body part, again toward the heart. The pressure can be increased or decreased, depending on the tone of the muscles and the depth of penetration desired. Both hands may be used alternately to grasp, lift, and gently squeeze the muscles and tissue. As the tissue slides out from under one hand, it is picked up by the other. Often the hands move in a circular motion toward each other as this is done. The same motion can be employed using only one hand, the two thumbs, or a thumb and a finger. When rolling is used,

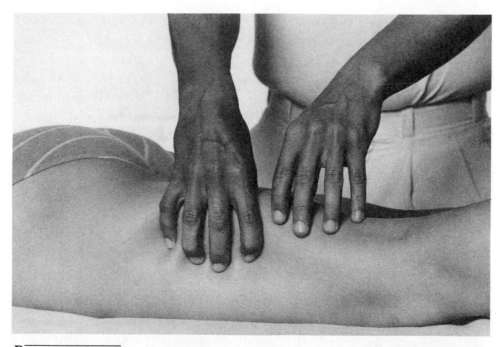

Petrissage: kneading thigh and buttocks. Always work in the direction of the heart.

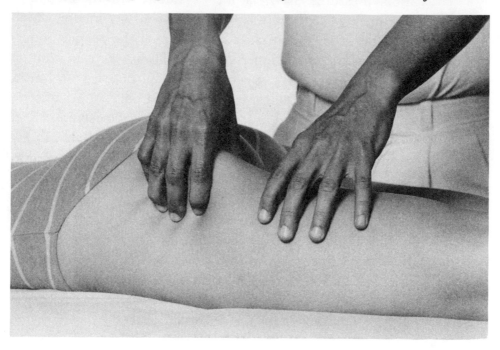

the muscle and tissues are grasped and rolled around the bone while the hands move slowly along the body part.

Petrissage improves circulation by stimulating blood flow to the heart on a deeper level than effleurage. By moving the tissues deeply, it assists in the removal of fluids that cause swelling and increases the removal and elimination of cellular waste materials and toxins. Nerve endings are stimulated and the tone of the entire body is improved.

This stroke provides an excellent warmup for muscle action and is particularly beneficial for athletes, dancers, and gymnasts prior to competition or performance and can eliminate soreness and stiffness if used afterward. By imitating the muscles' own movements, it invigorates, cleanses, and tones. It is particularly useful for the extremities, abdomen, and back.

- *Friction* is performed with the thumb, fingertips, palm, or heel of the hand, depending on the size and shape of the body part being massaged. It consists of small circular movements of various pressures. *Superficial friction* is done with the fingers or hand moving over the surface of the skin. In *deep friction,* which causes the superficial tissues to move over the deeper underlying ones, the practitioner's hand is always kept in contact with the client's body. Deep friction can be used around a joint or to get into the center or broadest part of the muscle.

Joints are mobilized as a result of friction's loosening effect on the connective tissues. *Transverse friction* can stretch a shortened muscle by loosening the fibers and can strengthen a joint. This technique is performed by moving across the muscle fibers and is often used in sports massage. *Rectilinear friction* is done in the same direction as the fibers or by following the long axis of the limb. It can be useful when the muscle is too tight or sensitive to be worked on circularly or transversely. Adhesions and scar tissues are broken down, and swelling around a joint will decrease as deposits and waste products are dispersed and toxins are absorbed.

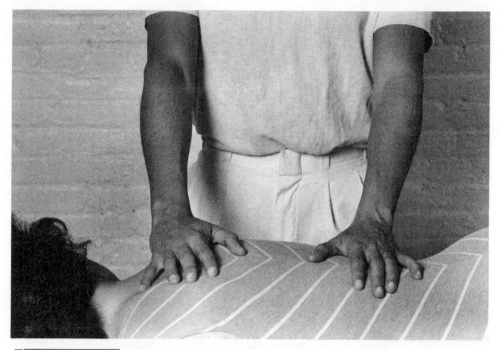

Friction to the back. Rocking back and forth relieves tired muscles.

The benefits of friction are more localized than the other strokes, and it generally has a deeper effect. Stiff joints, edema, sciatica, rheumatism, sprains, paralysis, fractures, and muscle problems all respond well to this technique.

- *Tapotement,* a French word for "percussion," is accomplished with short, rapid strokes on the body with the hands or fingers and can be done in any direction. Many different percussion techniques have been used, but the basic four are:

1. hacking—performed with the outside edge of the hand
2. tapping—applied with the fingertips, either lightly or firmly
3. cupping (or clapping)—done with cupped palms, with the fingers held together
4. beating—either with loose or tight fists

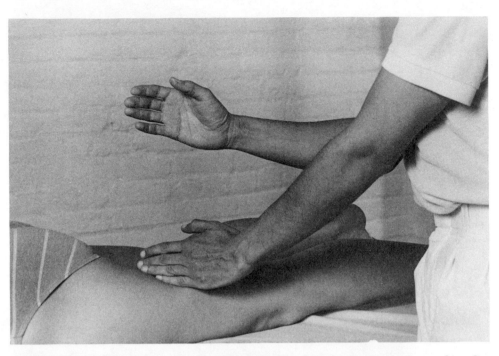

Tapotement means "percussion." While alternating hands, firmly apply rapid strokes using the palms or sides of the hands—really loosens up that muscle!

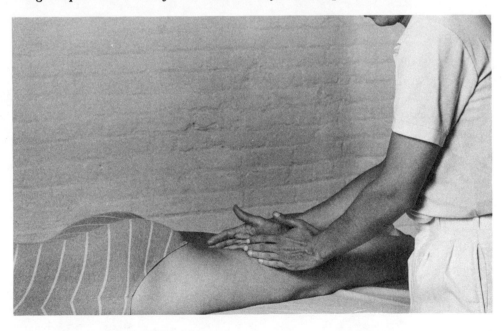

Tapotement is an underrated stroke. Its effect on the body is profound, stimulating the deeper structures and increasing circulation and metabolic rate. Tapotement breaks up congestion in the lungs when it is performed on the chest area and upper back. Cramps and muscle tensions respond well to percussive strokes, and muscle tone can be improved. It also stimulates muscle contraction and nerve sensibility, creating an excitatory response. If the stroke is continued for more than ten to fifteen seconds, however, it may result in overstimulation of the nerves and tissues. If continued for more than a minute, an exhausting effect can be produced. Hyperactive children can often be calmed by exhausting their nervous and muscular activity in this way.

■ *Vibration* is often a difficult stroke to master, involving as it does a definite rhythm and steady coordination. It is performed by placing the hand or fingertips on the body and creating a trembling, shaking sensation. The hands may move continuously or from time to time over the body. Vibration can be combined with effleurage and petrissage, making it a "running" vibratory stroke.

Heavier tissues such as on the back, abdomen, and legs are best vibrated with the hand, while the fingers may be used for thinner areas, such as the head, face, neck, and sides of the spine.

As in tapotement, the nerves are stimulated and the length of time determines whether the effect will be stimulating, relaxing, or exhausting.

Vibration on the face and head can relieve headaches and sinus conditions. Vibration stimulates contraction of the muscles, circulation, glandular secretion, and peristalsis in the bowels.

In various therapeutic settings, vibration is often accomplished through the use of machines. This can be effective, but the operator has to be fully aware of the intensity of the vibration to know how long to use it.

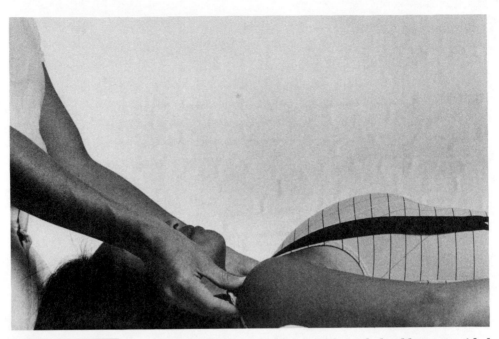

Vibration applied to the neck muscles. Headaches and tired shoulders are aided by the release of tight neck muscles.

All Swedish massage strokes require evenness, rhythm, and the proper use of body weight by the practitioner. A skilled masseuse or masseur uses his or her own body weight vigorously; if not, fatigue can easily result.

Swedish massage is generally done with the client lying on a table, although parts of the body may be massaged with the person in a sitting position. The use of the table is a historical development stemming from the practice of massage on injured soldiers in hospitals. It is also advantageous to the posture of the practitioner. The table should be the proper height for easy stance and sufficient leverage, and it should be flexible enough to accommodate the pressures of the various strokes. A padded surface will provide flexibility as well as comfort for the client. Plenty of clean sheets and towels should be on hand to cover and support the client's body. For example, when a client is in the prone position, a rolled-up towel should be placed beneath the ankles to relieve strain and pressure on the knee joints.

Draping the client properly is an important part of the massage. A sheet covering the table and hanging over the sides is used to wrap the person from either side, providing comfort and warmth during the session, since body temperature drops in areas that are not being massaged. The client is advised to keep his or her eyes closed, and little or no talking should take place, thus encouraging the person to relax completely and focus inwardly.

A lubricant is usually used, except in cases in which deep friction is needed. Oil is the most common lubricant, although cream is often used and occasionally talc, which is generally preferred by Russians. The lubricant provides a smooth surface on which to execute the strokes and prevents skin burns, jerky movements, and pulling the hairs on the body. It also promotes suppleness of the skin. Effleurage is a good stroke with which to administer and spread the oil. It should not be poured directly on the client from the bottle; oil or cream should be warmed first in the practitioner's hands before application.

Moist heat packs are sometimes used to warm and relax the muscles prior to massage. This allows the practitioner to get to the deeper structures in a shorter period of time.

Emphasis is placed on cleanliness, neatness, courtesy, and professionalism at all times. Massage therapists usually wear a white coat while working, are neatly groomed, maintain an air of efficiency, and are good listeners. Books and charts should be readily at hand, both to check various conditions and to educate the client.

Swedish massage techniques are easily applied to many areas of one's own body and can be used to relieve pain, soreness, stiffness, and tension. Self-massage is particularly beneficial prior to exercise and should be done vigorously to warm up the muscles.

■ Education, Training, and Careers

Massage therapists come from all walks of life and are generally earthy, caring people who enjoy working with their hands. Swedish massage is taught at many schools in the United States and abroad.

Different states and countries have varying licensing laws, and some do not require a license to practice as a professional. In those states that do, attendance at a state-approved school and successful completion of a state examination are mandatory. In the United States, there are presently eleven states that require licensing (see list at the end of this chapter).

The American Massage Therapy Association (AMTA) is an international organization of massage therapists. There are chapters in thirty-six of the states in this country and in various countries throughout the world. The AMTA publishes a quarterly journal, sponsors conferences, and provides general information.

One of the major schools of Swedish massage is The Swedish Institute in New York City, founded by Captain Theodore Melander, a native of Sweden, in 1904.

Approximately thirty-five schools in the United States and Canada have AMTA-approved curricula. (Not all of these schools are state approved, nor do all state-approved schools have an AMTA-approved curriculum.) The minimum number of hours of training required by these schools is five hundred. The number of hours vary from school to school, however, with the maximum number being about fifteen hundred. Non–AMTA-approved schools may require fewer hours. Students learn anatomy, physiology, pathology, cardiopulmonary resuscitation (CPR), first aid, Swedish massage techniques, medical massage, and adjunctive therapies, such as Eastern systems of bodywork and ethical and business practices.

The career possibilities for Swedish massage therapists are endless. In addition to independent practice, a large percentage of graduates of Swedish massage schools become practitioners in health clubs, spas, and resorts. Other opportunities can be found aboard cruise ships, in beauty salons, and in holistic health centers. As the specific medical and therapeutic benefits are becoming more recognized, jobs are opening in other health professions, such as with chiropractors, who realize that massage therapy can help make their work easier and longer lasting. Massage is also becoming more prominent in the sports world as more people have begun participating in various types of amateur athletics. Massage has always been used in boxing, but it is now becoming part of other individual and team sports. Also, as corporations are beginning to recognize the importance of preventive health care and stress reduction for their employees, more and more opportunities are opening in the corporate sector.

■ How to Locate a Practitioner

Licensed practitioners can be located by contacting your state or regional chapter of the AMTA, local schools of massage, and holistic health centers.

■ States with Massage Laws

Arkansas
State Board Therapy Technology
Martha Farmers, President
103 Trivista, Left
Hot Springs 71901
Education requirements—1250 hours; state board written and practical examination.

Florida
Department of Professional Regulation
Board of Massage, Bill Lemocks
130 N. Monroe St.
Tallahassee 32301 (904) 487-2520
Education requirements—completion of a course of study at a state-approved massage school or of an apprenticeship of 1700 hours of prescribed study; state board written and practical examination.

Hawaii
Board of Massage
Department of Commerce and Consumer Affairs
Professional and Vocational Licensing Division
Box 3469, 1010 Richard St.
Honolulu 96801
Education requirements—written and practical examination; examination can be waived if applicant holds similar license in another state; apprenticeship.

Nebraska
Department of Health
Bureau of Examining
Box 95007, State Office Building
Lincoln 68509 (402) 471-2115
Education requirements—600 hours at approved school; apprenticeship of one year.

New Hampshire
Louise Brackett, License Coordinator
Department of Health Facilities Administration
Hazen Drive
Concord 03301 (603) 271-4592
Education requirements—graduation from recognized school with not less than 500 hours of instruction; reciprocity for other state licenses with equal or greater requirements.

New York
State Board of Massage
Judy E. Hall, Ph.D., Executive Secretary
Cultural Education Center, Room 3025
Albany 12230 (518) 474-3866
Education requirements—graduation from massage school with not less than 500 hours.

North Dakota
North Dakota Massage Board
Albert E. Dahlgrer
508 21st Ave. So.
Fargo 58103
Education requirements—graduation from AMTA-approved school with 1000 hours of study.

Ohio
Angela Albert, Chief Licensure
The State Medical Board
65 So. Front St., Suite 510
Columbus 43215
Education requirements—graduation from approved school of massage with 250 hours of instruction.

Oregon
Massage Technicians Licensing Board
Peggy G. Smith, Executive Secretary
Department of Human Resources, Health Division
Box 231, 1400 SW 5th Ave.
Portland 97207
Education requirements—written, oral, and practical examination; reciprocity.

Rhode Island
State of Rhode Island and Providence Plantations
Professional Regulation
Department of Health
Robert W. McClanaghan, Administrator
Davis St., Cannon Building
Providence 02908
Education requirements—graduation from AMTA-approved school or equivalent.

Washington
State of Washington
Division of Professional Licensing
Box 9649
Olympia 98504 (206) 753-0776
Education requirements—written, oral and practical examination.

NOTE: Many cities and counties regulate the practice of massage with massage ordinances. Inquire at the city hall or county court house in the city or county that you plan to practice in for any massage regulations.

FOUR
REFLEXOLOGY/FOOT
MASSAGE

■ What Is Reflexology?

Reflexology or zone therapy is the stimulation of areas under the skin in order to improve the functioning of specific body parts. Reflexology can be divided into two general types. The first, which can be thought of as macroreflexology, deals with reflex areas throughout the entire body. Acupressure and acupuncture are the best-known examples of macroreflexology. The second type can be called microreflexology. The entire body is the macrosystem. Small, compact areas of the body are microsystems. This chapter is concerned with microsystems such as the feet, hands, and ears.

■ Benefits of Reflexology

Reflexology has a number of objectives:

- improved nerve and blood supply

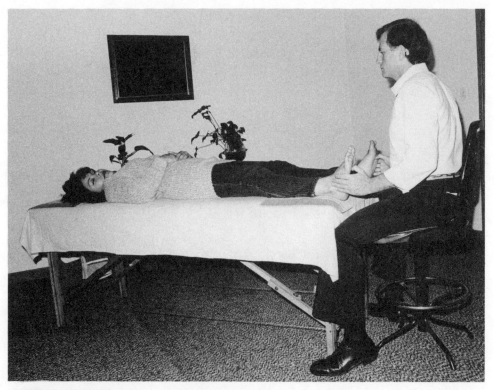

Expert Bill Flocco in his California office, working on feet.

- overall reduction of the effects of stress
- reduction, and sometimes actual elimination, of aches and pains
- improved circulation in the area being reflexed, as well as the entire body
- prevention of illness and maintenance of an optimal state of health
- normalization of body functions, such as lowering the activity of the thyroid or increasing the activity of the pancreas
- elimination of stress-related imbalances, which can affect every organ, gland, and structure of the body

Reflexology is particularly suitable for individuals who desire and need bodywork but have inhibitions about removing their clothes, which certain forms of bodywork require. There are also many individuals who do not like to be touched on the torso. For such individuals, reflexology is an acceptable and gratifying bodywork technique.

■ Background and History of Reflexology

Many people have contributed to the basic principles of reflexology as it is practiced on feet, hands, and ears. Reflex areas have also been found on the abdomen, back, arm, leg, neck, scalp, face, nose, tongue, and wrist.

Ear reflexology was first used by the ancient Chinese. In 1967, Dr. Nogier of France discovered the similarity between the shape of the outer ear and the shape of the fetus and the corresponding locations of reflexes. As a result of this finding, the Chinese have acknowledged Dr. Nogier as the father of auricular (ear) reflexology, which has since been extensively researched by both the French and the Chinese.

Hand reflexology was also first used in China. A different system has been developed in America, based on the zone theory of Dr. William H. Fitzgerald. Other pioneers include Dr. Edwin F. Bowers, Dr. George Starr White, and Mildred Carter.

Foot reflexology is the most commonly practiced form of reflexology in the United States and Europe. Different systems have been developed in China, Japan, and India. In the United States, it was first developed in the early 1900s by Dr. Fitzgerald, Dr. Joseph Riley, and Eunice Ingham, who, using Dr. Fitzgerald's zone theories, developed what is today known as reflexology.

■ Basic Philosophy and Principles of Reflexology

A *reflex* is defined as an "involuntary response to a stimulus." Reflexology utilizes specific reflex points—parts of the body that, when stimulated, produce a reflex response in another part. The system is based on the principle that the stimulus-response reflex is conducted through neural pathways in the body that activate the body's biochemical and electrochemical activities.

Reflexes depend on an intact neural pathway between the point of stimulation and the responding organ, muscle, or gland. This pathway is called a reflex arc and includes a sensory receptor, a sensory neuron, the relaxation centers in the brain and spinal cord, efferent neurons, and a muscle or gland.

The use of neural pathways to produce a stimulus-response reflex is the basis for several other bodywork systems, including acupressure, myotherapy, and polarity. Reflexology differs from these systems, as reflexology specifically applies to reflexes in the feet and hands.

There are three major systems of reflexology: Western theory, Eastern theory, and zone theory.

Western theory maintains that a large number of nerve endings are found in the hands, feet, and ears. When an imbalance occurs somewhere in the body, chemical congestion takes place between the nerve endings and the corresponding reflex points in the hands, feet, and ears that correspond to the specific body part with an imbalance. By placing proper pressure on the reflex areas, the congestion is dissipated. The electrochemical energy of the nerves can then flow freely again. This permits the restoration of harmony to the body part that was out of balance. This theory is applicable to foot, hand, and ear reflexology.

Eastern theory maintains that energy pathways known as meridians run throughout the body. They are as thin as a thread and run up and down the body from head to toe as well as up and down the arms from fingers to chest. The theory further states that specific meridian points in the hands and feet correspond to particular areas and functions of the body.

When an imbalance occurs in a body part or a particular function of the body, an imbalance also occurs in the corresponding point on the hands and feet. With proper pressure, these reflex imbalances in the hands and feet are often eliminated, thus restoring harmony to the affected part of the body. As both hands and feet are completely reflexed, these points are affected in such a way as to eliminate the imbalances in the points as well as the corresponding body part. Meridians are found in the hands and feet but not in the ears. Consequently, Eastern theory applies to foot and hand reflexology, but not to ear reflexology.

Zone theory was the forerunner of hand and foot reflexology as practiced today in the United States. Dr. William H. Fitzgerald discovered that by putting pressure on one part of the body, an anesthetic effect could be produced in another part. He postulated the existence of ten zones, each corresponding to a finger and toe, which run vertically up and down the leg, torso, neck, and head. These zones are joined in the chest area by corresponding zones running up the fingers and arms. The big toes and the thumbs are zone number 1. When someone has an imbalance anywhere in this zone, there will probably be an imbalance in zone number 1 in the hands and feet. By applying pressure to zone number 1 in the hands and feet, the imbalance elsewhere in zone number 1 of the body often is eliminated. Since the outer ear is found only in zone number 5, the zone theory does not seem to apply to ear reflexology.

Reflex areas can provide clues to possible imbalances elsewhere in the body in a number of ways. Most commonly, tender spots discovered while reflexing indicate an imbalance in the corresponding part of the body. When such tenderness is found, extra time should be spent reflexing the area in order to dissipate the congestion. The longer the imbalance has existed, the longer it usually takes to eliminate it. Sore, tender areas may be relieved in minutes or may take months to alleviate.

Other indications of possible imbalances in the body are one or more of the following in the reflex area: redness and other color irregularities, patches of dry or oily skin, itchiness, sensitivity when no reflexing is being done, temperature irregularities, and electrochemical irregularities; however temperature and electrical irregularities require sensitive measuring devices that are beyond the scope of popular forms of reflexology.

These symptoms do not always mean that something is out of balance

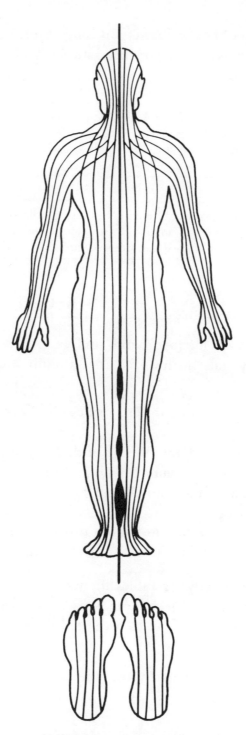

Each line represents a zone. If imbalance is found in one area, it may be caused by an area in a corresponding zone.

elsewhere in the body. A variety of other causes could contribute to the signals, such as a toe having been stubbed, a hand muscle strained, or an ear scratched.

IMPORTANT: Before beginning a session, make sure your nails are short and smooth for comfort's sake. If working on feet, check for corns, calluses, ingrown toenails, or any area that might cause discomfort through direct contact.

Reflexology instructors caution against using reflexology for diagnostic purposes or prescribing anything or treating a specific condition, unless you are a properly trained and licensed medical practitioner.

■ Reflexology Techniques

Techniques vary for foot, hand, and ear reflexology. In hand and foot reflexology, the "inchworm" (or "thumb walk") is the primary technique used.

1. Place your thumb flat, print side down, on the area being reflexed.
2. Roll forward onto the tip of the thumb to make a 90-degree angle between your thumb and the area being reflexed. The pressure from your thumb provides the maximum reflexive effectiveness.
3. Slide the thumb forward a little, flatten it, and then roll up onto the tip again.

This movement clearly resembles the way an inchworm moves.

The "hook and pull" technique is used primarily on the hands yet can also be used on the feet to a limited degree. It is also known as the grasp technique.

1. Place your fingertips on the part of the hand facing away from you.

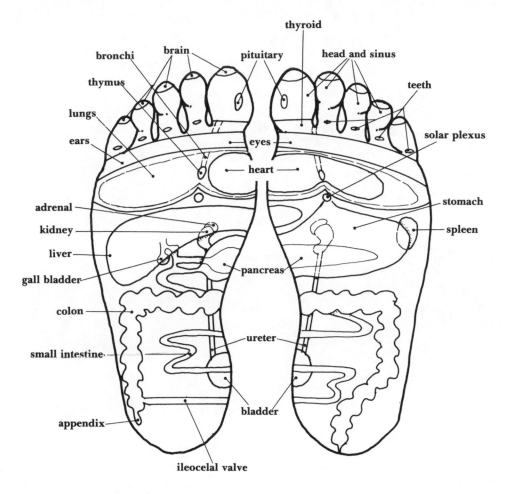

thyroid
brain
bronchi pituitary head and sinus
thymus teeth
lungs
ears eyes solar plexus
heart
adrenal stomach
kidney spleen
liver
gall bladder pancreas
colon
small intestine ureter
appendix bladder
ileocelal valve

2. Pull your fingertips toward your palm as if grasping the tissue in your hand.

3. With the tips of your fingers on the part to be reflexed, pull as if you are pulling toward yourself.

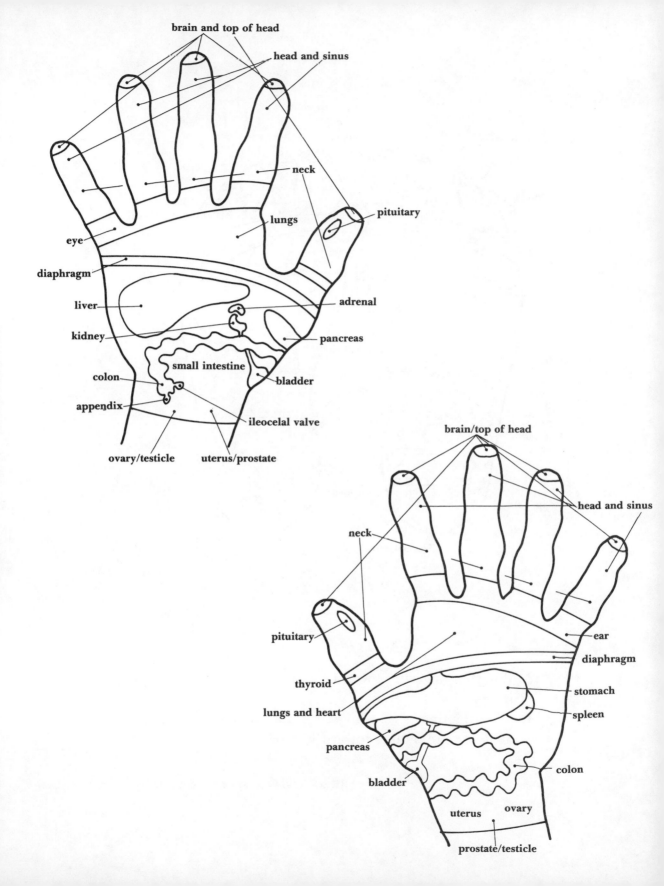

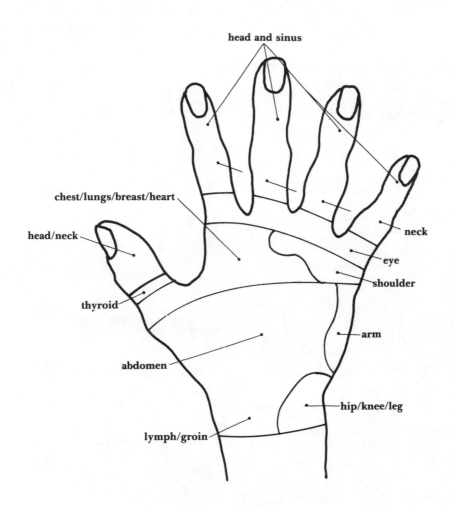

head and sinus

chest/lungs/breast/heart

head/neck

neck

eye

shoulder

thyroid

arm

abdomen

hip/knee/leg

lymph/groin

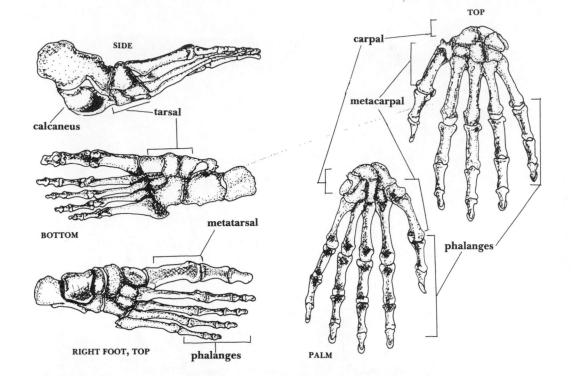

SIDE

calcaneus

tarsal

BOTTOM

metatarsal

RIGHT FOOT, TOP

phalanges

TOP

carpal

metacarpal

phalanges

PALM

phalanges

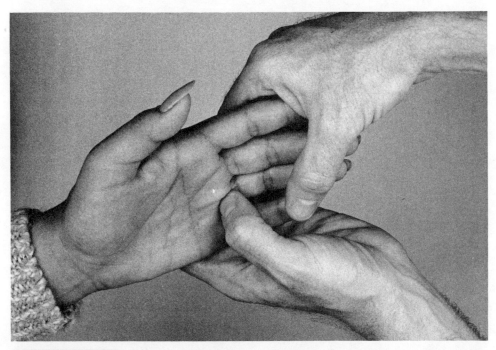

The "inchworm" or "thumbwalk" technique. Photo by Jason Moss, courtesy of The Reflexology Workshop.

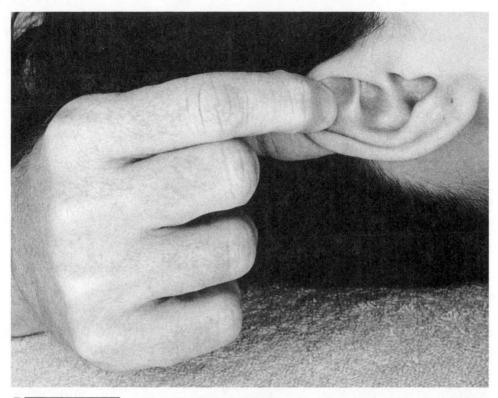

Reflex for the ear. Press in as shown with firm pressure and hold for ten seconds.

Ear reflexology is done primarily by rubbing various points on the ear. Sometimes pressure is maintained as part of the ear is held between the tips of the index finger and the thumb. Sometimes light pressure is applied with one of the fingernails being placed on a specific reflex point.

There are many different techniques for reflexology, but these are the basic ones for the hands, feet, and ears. Although it is possible to get an idea about these techniques from a book, there is no substitute for in-class, hands-on instruction.

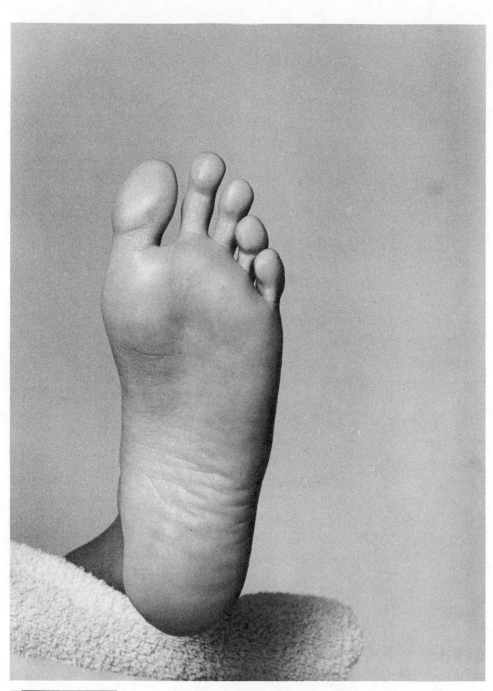

The foot can tell the story of what is going on in your body.

82   MASSAGE TECHNIQUES

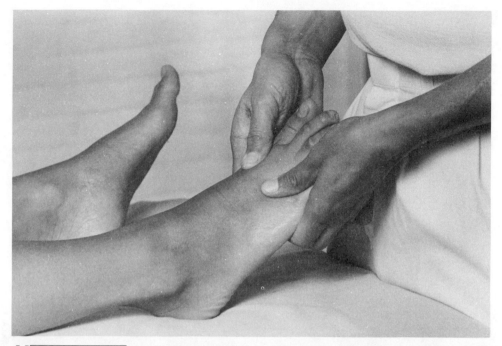

Massaging the feet. Hold foot with both hands. Wiggle the fingers down the front of the foot from toes to ankles. Then rotate thumbs in a circular motion over the entire foot. Revitalizing massage oil may be applied to entire foot to reduce skin-to-skin friction.

Muscle squeeze to foot to relieve tension and increase circulation. Squeeze entire foot on both sides, applying firm pressure.

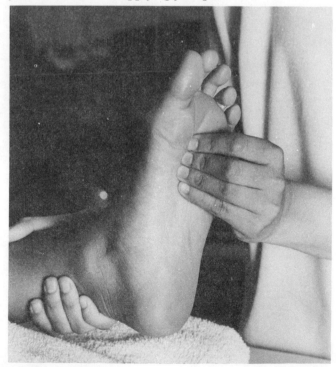

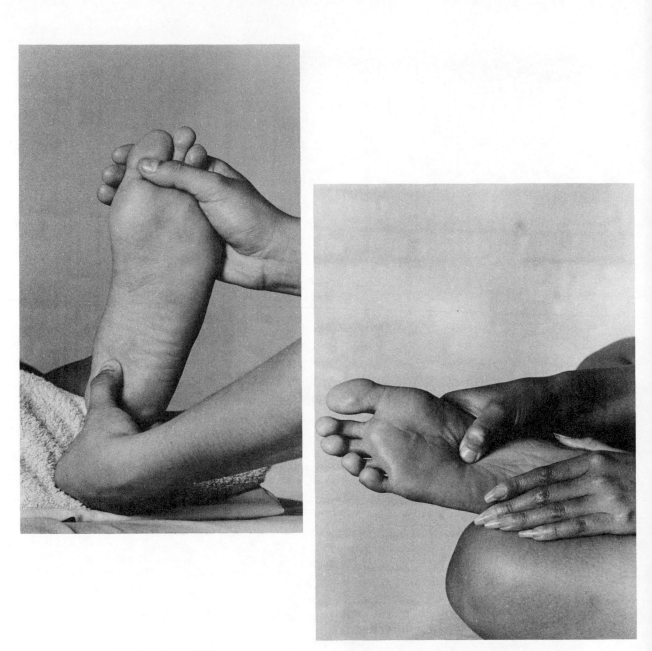

S̄ciatic nerve reflex to relieve hip and thigh pain. Using the knuckle of the index finger, press lightly in and hold for about five seconds.

R̄eflex to stomach.

84   MASSAGE TECHNIQUES

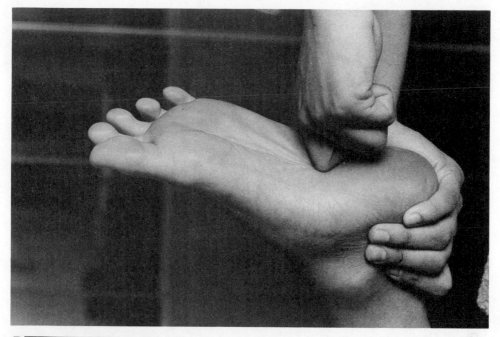

Reflex to small intestine.

Reflex to sex glands. Locate on the outside of the foot, just below the ankle. Press in firmly for about seven seconds. Then massage this area using small circular motions. Do this to both feet.

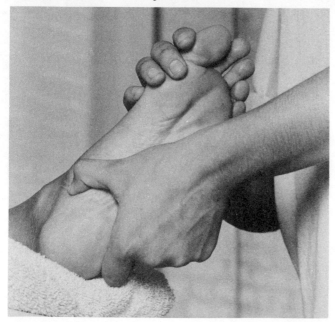

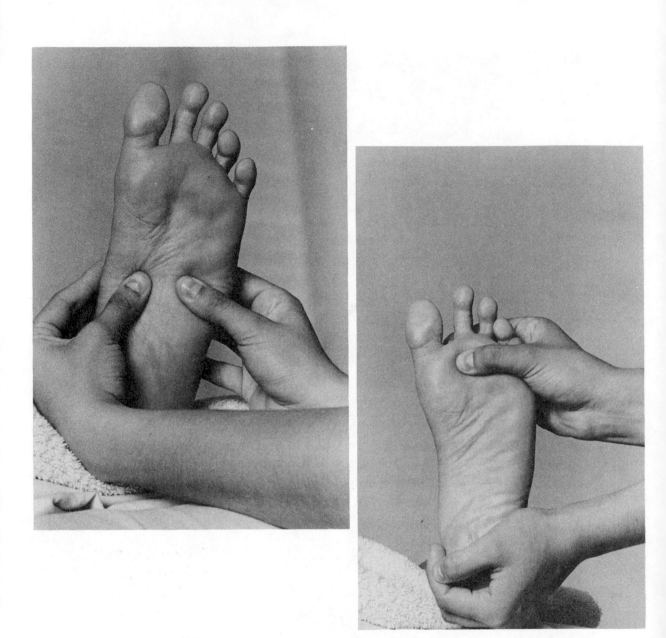

Reflex to colon. Use both hands to massage horizontally in opposite directions. Begin in center and then move to outside of foot.

Stimulating the thyroid gland reflex to increase energy. Press in for seven seconds. Repeat three times.

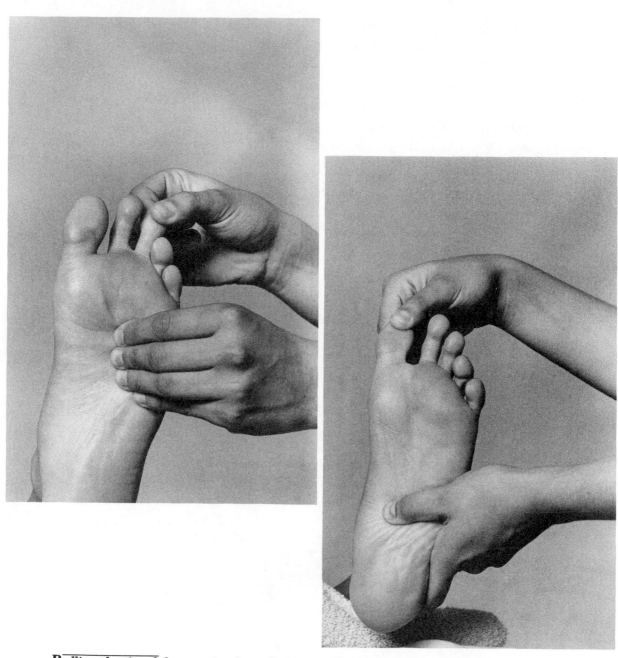

Pulling the tip of the toe stimulates the sinus reflex for breathing. Hold the tip in your fingers and gently rotate toe. Then press the tips from the tops and hold for ten seconds. Repeat three times on each toe.

REFLEXOLOGY/FOOT MASSAGE   87

It is important to underscore that reflexology is done with the hands. The use of implements is discouraged. While most people use powder on the feet and hands, some use oil. Powder absorbs perspiration, gives a smooth texture for moving easily over the surface of the skin, and allows for a firm grip. A common approach is to use powder on the feet during the treatment and then to rub aromatic warm oils on the feet for a few minutes after treatment. Some people also use a warm foot bath at the beginning of the session. For a relaxing and healthful treat, try soaking your feet in a hot tub or using a foot bath/massager, such as the Foot Fixer by Clairol. This relaxes and soothes tired, aching feet; feels good; and helps relax the rest of the body. By keeping your feet free of pain, relaxed, and in good condition, you are helping to facilitate good health in the other parts of your body.

Most professional reflexologists work on people as they are sitting in a reclining chair or lying on a massage table. However, for the lay

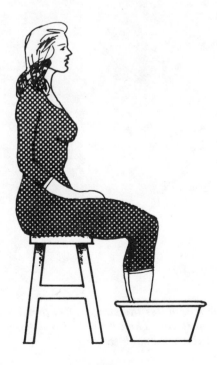

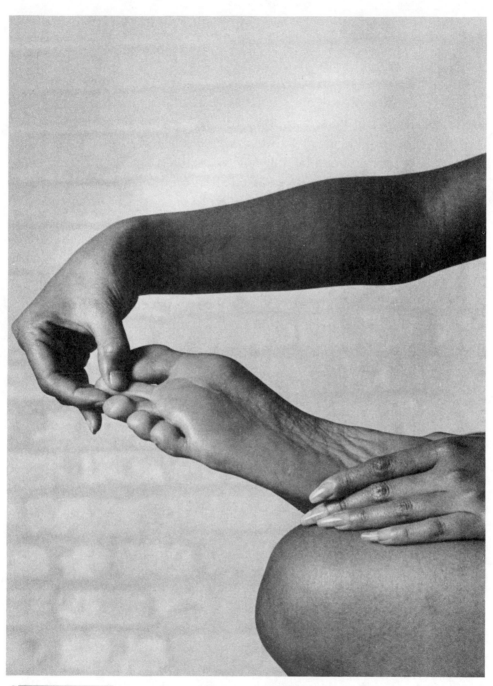

Self-massage, sinus breathing reflex.

person, reflexology is easily done with the recipient lying on the floor or on a bed, with the feet over the edge. Reflexology for the hands and ears can be administered in almost any position.

One of the best aspects of reflexology is that you can use it on yourself as easily as on someone else. It is, in fact, one of the only bodywork modalities that can be self-applied to balance your entire body.

With slight modifications, all the reflexology techniques that can be used on someone else can be done on yourself. In fact, hand reflexology is much easier to perform on yourself than on another person. This is because you are able to hold your own hand very steady, whereas when working on another person, the hand is often flexible, making the treatment more difficult.

CAUTION: Reflexology should not be done in an area where there is a fracture, a torn ligament or tendon, or excruciating pain. It also is not advisable to attempt reflexology during pregnancy. If there are varicose veins in the lower leg, do not include that area in your treatment.

■ Education, Training, and Career Development

Most reflexology training programs are for beginners who want to use reflexology on themselves, their family, and their friends. These programs usually last for from six months to two years, depending on the individual's background. Some people who have experience in the field of bodywork or have a highly sensitive natural touch can, with a few weekends of intensive training and a good deal of supervised practice, become competent within a few months.

Two levels of certification are available in the field of reflexology: a certificate of completion and a certificate of competency. Most people who study reflexology for nonprofessional use receive a certificate of completion, which indicates that the individual has acquired rudimentary knowledge and some basic skills in the field. The extent of knowledge or skills is not specified. A certificate of competency, on the other hand, indicates that the person has completed a basic, intermediate, and advanced training program and has demonstrated specified knowledge and skills through written, oral, and applied examinations. Most schools provide training in foot reflexology only, although there are variations.

A wide range of career opportunities is available in reflexology. Most practitioners incorporate it with other health and healing modalities. Nurses, massage therapists, shiatsu practitioners, acupressurists, chiropractors, physical therapists, manicurists, and pedicurists are in a natural position to incorporate reflexology techniques into their work. Some people specialize in reflexology only and practice it on a part-time basis, treating perhaps five to ten clients a week.

The Reflexology Workshop in Los Angeles, California, is the only training program in the United States that provides training in the three major reflexology areas: feet, hands, and ears. The workshop's director, Bill Flocco, teaches throughout the western United States. Laura Norman and Associates, Reflexologists, provide training in New York City. Other schools in the United States are found in Florida; a prominent one is the International Institute of Reflexology in St. Petersburg, Florida. There are also schools in England and Germany.

■ How to Locate a Reflexology Practitioner

There are several ways to find a certified reflexologist:

1. In larger cities, look in the Yellow Pages of your telephone directory.
2. Look in health publications that deal with bodywork, nutrition, and other forms of natural health care.
3. Check with local health-food and metaphysical bookstores.
4. Contact a reflexology school in your area.
5. Contact Bill Flocco, Reflexology Workshop.

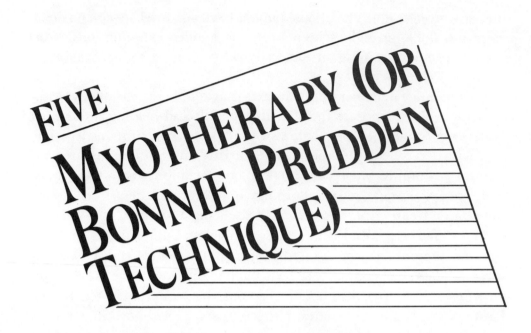

FIVE
MYOTHERAPY (OR BONNIE PRUDDEN TECHNIQUE)

■ What Is Myotherapy?

Myotherapy is a system for the treatment of muscular pain and dysfunction. It is used to remedy flare-ups of trigger points—irritable spots in the muscles that can be caused at birth or through accidents, strain, or disease—that cause pain and muscle spasm, without the use of drugs or surgical techniques. Unlike the pressure points or techniques in acupressure, the trigger points in myotherapy are different in each person. Myotherapy, through the use of pressure alone, is able to eliminate the spasms caused by trigger-point flare-ups. Bonnie Prudden believes that 95 percent of all chronic pain is muscular in origin. She is a true pioneer who has developed a revolutionary technique of pain relief that has earned widespread medical endorsement.

■ Benefits of Myotherapy

Myotherapy can be used to eliminate pain in any part of the body.

It is also beneficial in the elimination of headaches, dizziness, bursitis, numbness in fingers and toes, arthritis, menstrual cramps, spastic colon, heartburn, and asthmatic pain, as well as other sources of discomfort. Today many doctors are beginning to use myotherapy as a diagnostic test. That use has been pioneered by Dr. Desmond R. Tivey. If the patient with chronic back pain gets rid of it in one or two sessions, there isn't much sense in putting him or her through expensive tests. However, it is wise to caution that if myotherapy doesn't work, tests and/or consultation with a physician may be the next step. The Stockbridge Institute claims to have a 95 percent success rate with myotherapy patients.

■ Background and History of Myotherapy

Myotherapy was developed in 1976 by Bonnie Prudden. As she describes her experience, she was mountain climbing with friends and awoke one morning with a very painful and stiff neck. She had had a recurring pain sporadically for years, since being thrown from a bucking horse. A physician who was a member of the climbing party took one look at her lopsided head and suggested that she not continue her climb. He then pressed the back of her neck so hard, according to Prudden, that "my knees buckled." She had a knot in her neck, and he kept pressing. When he stopped applying pressure, the knot was gone and her head appeared to be in a straight position. Best of all, the pain was gone and she was able to continue her climb.

Janet Travell, M.D., was the pioneer in the medical discipline labeled trigger-point injection therapy. The process involved probing with a finger until a tender spot was found, indicating the presence of a trigger point. The trigger point was then injected with a solution, usually of saline and procaine. Dr. Travell followed the injection with a gentle passive stretch and finished with a cooling spray of fluorimethane.

Bonnie Prudden's system of myotherapy differs from Dr. Travell's trigger-point injection therapy primarily in that there are no injections. While working with a client who complained of a painful tennis elbow,

Prudden marked the arm near the trigger point and applied pressure with her thumb. The response was pain. She then probed up and down the entire arm, pressing trigger points as she located them. Fifteen minutes later the client was feeling no pain and the elbow had full range of movement. She thereby discovered that properly applied pressure, rather than injections, could be used effectively to eliminate pain caused by a trigger point.

In 1978, Prudden founded the Institute for Physical Fitness and Myotherapy. Recognized as a foremost authority on physical fitness, she has conducted extensive research on the physical fitness of American children and was a member of the President's Council on Physical Fitness and Sports in the 1950s. The author of numerous books and articles on exercise and health, she has also produced several films on the subject as well as an eighty-minute audiovisual cassette, *Myotherapy: Pain-free Living*. Her book *Pain Erasure the Bonnie Prudden Way* has been widely read and acclaimed.

■ Basic Principles and Philosophy of Myotherapy

Myotherapy involves what is known medically as trigger points. Basically, a trigger point is a highly irritable spot in a muscle. Many theories exist about how trigger points are caused. According to Bonnie Prudden, birth trauma, falls suffered in childhood, certain diseases, poor posture, sports injuries or strains, occupational hazards, and even the stress of daily living can cause the formation of trigger points.

Some trigger points develop deep in the muscle and lie dormant for years, then flare up as a result of emotional or physical stress. When a flare-up occurs, the result is a painful muscle spasm. Spasms may also occur as reflexes. That is, when the spasm sent by the nervous system reaches a certain area, it may further tighten an already present spasm in that area. This she calls splinting, or the spasm-pain-spasm cycle.

The objective of myotherapy is to stop the muscle spasm and end the pain. This is accomplished through the application of pressure to the trigger point that is causing the problem. Spasms in the muscles, in addition to causing pain, also cause misalignment. Once the spasm has been stopped and the muscle has relaxed, realignment of the muscle occurs. The muscle is then reeducated to perform normally through gentle stretching exercises. Myotherapy works both on pain incurred through recent injuries and on chronic pain.

■ Myotherapy Techniques

Myotherapy is usually done on a massage table. It employs the use of a bodo (a wooden dowel attached to wooden handles, which comes in three sizes. The smallest is used on hands and feet; the other two are helpful in self-treatment in myotherapy). Also used is fluorimethane, a cooling spray. According to myotherapy specialists, this helps speed the pain-relief process. The spray is only available by prescription. As an alternative, refer to the section on hydrotherapy in which ice is used as an anesthetic (p. 124). Ice cubes applied to a painful area may prove helpful, as cold travels along nerve pathways faster than pain. The autonomic nervous system does not get the message of pain and thus the feeling of pain is suppressed.

Tracing paper is used when searching out trigger points (for future reference). A black pen is used to trace the trigger points, showing the muscles to be treated. This becomes a map to guide the myotherapist for easy future location of trigger points on an individual.

Depending on the amount of pressure needed and the location of the trigger point, fingers, knuckles, and elbows are used. You are, in fact, searching for and neutralizing the trigger points. After finding the first one, search and move along the muscle at approximately one-inch intervals. Each time you locate one, rest and press for about seven seconds. Keep moving along until you find a trigger point. Trigger points may express themselves through tenderness or even the sensation of pain. The first session is usually the most painful; however, the treatment gets less painful with time. Though seven seconds of pressure is average for most trigger points, the sensation may be more intense

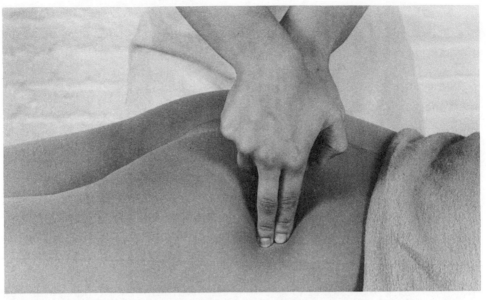

Use your fingers to locate a painful spot. Press down lightly. This technique releases tension in the gluteal muscles and may be helpful in eliminating menstrual cramps.

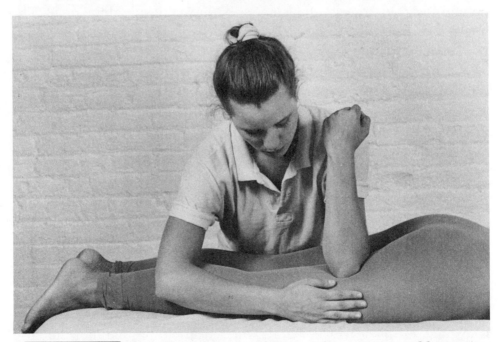

Locating and erasing a trigger point in the leg to relieve cramps and leg tension. Apply slight pressure to area just below buttocks.

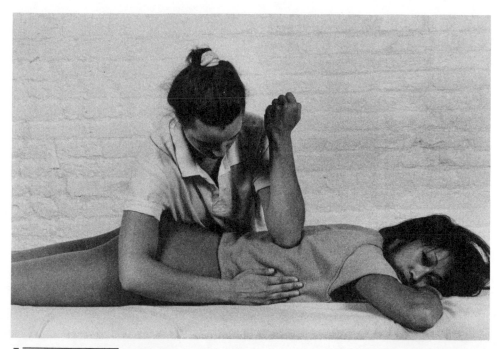

Locating and using elbow to erase trigger point in lower back. Lean in (slightly at first) while applying pressure with elbow.

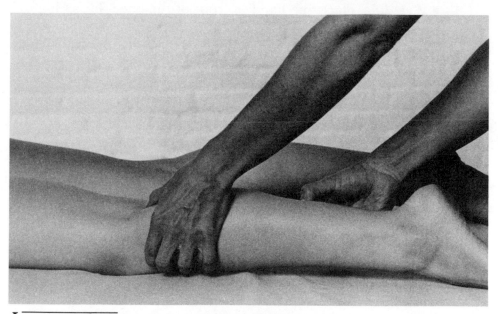

Locating and erasing a trigger point in the leg.

in the face and the head, so in those cases, use only four or five seconds of pressure.

Taking the entire approach to the body, myotherapists may also recommend effective therapeutic exercises. One very important concept in Bonnie Prudden's technique is continual or repetitious stimulation of a pressure point. That is, working over a number of sessions will ultimately bring relief, as opposed to working in just one simple session.

As a preventive measure, matrix holdouts are especially important for the athlete. Matrix holdouts are areas that are always tender, even when the subject no longer feels pain. They should be checked before any competition to prevent a spasm from the trigger point from occurring during a game.

Myotherapy is one of the most developed scientific approaches obtainable today to keep the body free of pain and in a state of good health. This is true because of the high caliber of Prudden's system and the certified myotherapists she trains.

■ Self-help Exercises

- *Knee lift* Place one hand in front of the knee; lift as high as possible. This strengthens arms and stretches the back. Lift each leg a few times. Do 4 repetitions on each side, alternating legs.
- *Free knee lift* Place your hands on the arms of the chair and, keeping the leg straight, bring the left knee as close to your nose as possible. Repeat with right knee.
- *Knee cross and kick* Keep the same body position and cross your knees without thinking about it. Slide your seat forward in the chair and lean back. Cross the left knee over the right and then alternate, then remove the knee and kick up as high as possible. Alternate legs.
- *Head roll* Next, sit relaxed in a chair or stand at ease. Let your head hang forward. Just relax and let it hang for five or six seconds. Check with the head, neck, and upper-lower back.

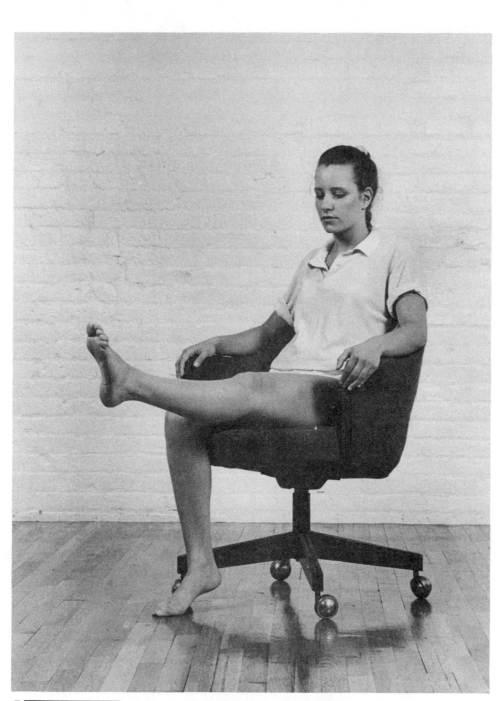

Leg exercise. Raise and extend the leg as far as possible.

Make sure that you feel no tension. Roll your head slowly to the right side. Next, roll your head slowly to the left, back and forth on the axis of your shoulder.

- *Heel lifts*   Place your feet flat on the floor and parallel. Keep the toes and the balls of the feet on the floor and raise the heels. Try to arch the foot and push the instep over the toes. Lower the foot and alternate the feet for several seconds.

- *Seat lift*   Place your hands in the arm of the chair close to the front and straighten your arms to lift your seat into the air. Lower slowly, taking five seconds to accomplish the descent. Start with 2 repetitions and work to 6.

- *Pushups*   Be sure your chair is anchored against the wall so it cannot slip. Be sure your feet are secure so you cannot slip. Stand back from the chair. Place your feet wide apart. Slowly lower your body into the let-down position, then push up and return to the standing position.

- *Knee bends*   Standing straight up, slowly bend to the ground with your knees, keeping your back straight. This exercise builds muscle and self-confidence.

- *Knee-to-nose kick*   Get down on all fours and bring the right knee as close to your nose as you can. Then stretch the leg back and up, at the same time raising the head. Repeat this on each side 4 times. This exercise strengthens the back muscles and the abdominal muscles.

As a general massage technique developed by Bonnie Prudden for baby massage or for baby exercise, lay both hands on the chest of the baby, move them outward to both sides, around the back to the center, following the outline of the baby's ribs, using both hands at the same time as if smoothing open the pages of a book. Repeat this 3 or 4 times. For further information or for more specific details on Bonnie Prudden's baby exercise technique, consult her or one of her professional or certified practitioners (see p. 101).

■ Training and Certification

Training in myotherapy can be obtained only at the Institute for Physical Fitness and Myotherapy. Certification is provided by the International Myotherapy Association. Training consists of 1,300 hours over a span of two years. An additional 45 hours are required every two years for recertification. The training includes the intensive study of anatomy and physiology. Since myotherapists do not diagnose, they will accept only patients referred by physicians or dentists.

■ Career Opportunities

Some myotherapists are hospital connected and work directly with outpatient services. Many work with dentists and doctors through referral. Most, however, are in private practice and are now located in twenty-three states.

■ How to Locate a Myotherapist

For information on how to find a certified myotherapist in your community, contact:

Institute for Physical Fitness and Myotherapy, Inc.
Box 205
Stockbridge, MA 01262
(413) 298-3066

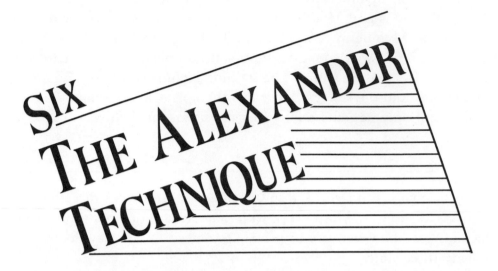

SIX
THE ALEXANDER TECHNIQUE

■ What Is the Alexander Technique?

By pinpointing inefficient neuromuscular patterns, the Alexander technique teaches us how to use our bodies appropriately and effectively as we go about our daily routines. It assists us in finding our center of balance and harmonizing with our environment. By making us more sensitive to the way we move, it teaches us a new way of thinking about and using our bodies so that we become more aware of unnecessary tension.

■ Benefits of the Alexander Technique

The basic aim of the Alexander technique is to help students become aware of how they move and to teach them to move with greater coordination and ease. As a consequence, everything we do becomes easier.

102

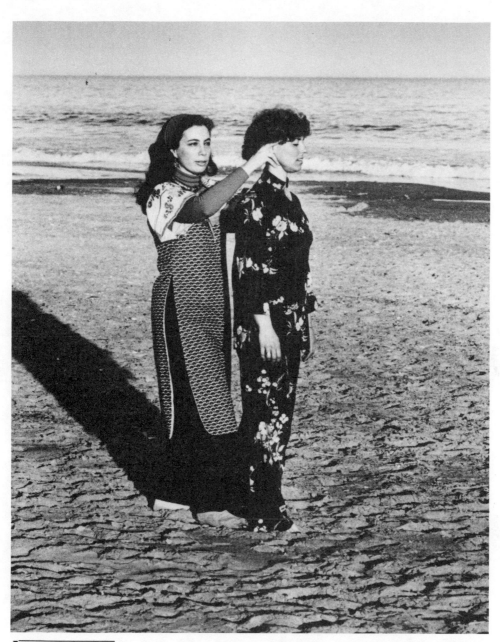

Illana Rubenfeld has teamed her extensive knowledge of the Alexander technique with *Moshe Feldenkrais* to develop the highly effective synergy method for combining movement, touch, and sensitivity.

The following are some of the specific benefits of the Alexander technique.

- We gain more flexibility, strength, and endurance through balanced muscle use.
- As compression within the body is relieved, our breathing becomes easier and fuller, and digestion and other internal functions improve because the organs and glands have enough space in which to function.
- Stress disorders respond very positively to Alexander work. As constricting muscles around the blood vessels relax, high blood pressure is reduced and the tendency to develop arteriosclerosis is lessened. Ulcers, colitis, bloating, constipation, and dysmenorrhea (menstrual troubles) respond favorably to the regular practice of the technique.
- Joint disorders such as rheumatoid and osteoarthritis; spinal disorders such as scoliosis, kyphosis, and lordosis; back pain; neuralgia; asthma and other respiratory disorders; muscular cramps and tics; and bruxism can all be relieved or eliminated through the Alexander technique. Surgery for muscular-skeletal problems such as slipped discs, scoliosis, and lumbosacral strain often can be avoided.
- Various psychosomatic and emotional disorders respond positively to the technique. Because the psychological and the physical are not separate aspects of the individual, we tend to reinforce our feelings with our bodies. When we experience anger, for example, our jaws tighten, our fists clench, and our muscles tend to tense. As we learn to balance our bodies, to employ the principles of use and inhibition, we release the muscular tensions associated with anger and can then redirect our energy to deal with the angry feelings in a productive way.
- Increased self-confidence and self-esteem are major benefits of the technique. We look better as our posture improves, and we learn to move more gracefully. People report more alert-

ness, cheerfulness, and positive feelings toward themselves, others, and life.
- Skills such as playing an instrument, dancing, singing, or watch repairing become more refined.

In practicing the Alexander technique, we learn to integrate thought and action. As we gain more strength, ease, balance, and freedom in our bodies, changing ingrained body habits, our mental and emotional spheres experience similar change.

■ Background and History of the Alexander Technique

The story of Frederick Matthias Alexander, the originator of the Alexander technique, is a unique and marvelous one in the world of self-discovery and healing. Born in 1869 in Tasmania, Alexander was an accomplished actor by the age of nineteen. Soon, however, he began to develop vocal problems and would suddenly lose his voice while on stage. When the problem became more serious and frequent, he was forced to curtail his acting engagements.

After seeking out many doctors, none of whom was able to help, he decided to take matters into his own hands and devised an ingenious system of mirrors whereby he could observe himself from many angles as he stood and spoke. As he adopted different stances, he noticed that he tended to pull his head backward and down ever so slightly. When he moved into a more balanced position, his voice returned.

He began to observe others and concluded that most people stood and moved in off-balance ways. He began to teach people how to regain proper use of their bodies—first actors, then singers, diplomats, teachers, musicians, and many others. Around the turn of the century, he traveled to London, where it became quite fashionable to have "Alexander lessons." Eventually he taught several of his pupils to teach his technique. He worked in both England and America, and through his pupils and his writings, his work spread throughout the world.

In recent years, his techniques have been used at four major educational institutions in England: The Royal College of Music, The Royal Academy of Dramatic Art, New College of Speech and Drama, and Guild Hall.

■ Basic Principles and Philosophy of the Alexander Technique

One of the key principles of the Alexander technique is that "use affects functioning." The way we use ourselves as we carry out an activity affects that activity. Our neuromuscular patterns are strong and tend to reinforce any continual activity, whether it is balanced or unbalanced.

Using our bodies well means using them in a properly integrated fashion. It means moving with maximum balance and coordination. This allows us to use only the amount of energy and the specific muscles necessary to carry out an activity.

In order to achieve good use, the spine should be long and the head should be balanced on top of the spine. This does not mean pushing ourselves into the military posture of chin up, shoulders back, as we are so often admonished. Because each individual is different and must learn to function within his or her own body structure, there is no "right" pose.

When the body is in balance and organized efficiently, we use it in a total way, since the body functions as an interconnected unit, one part balancing another. If this balance is not present, we may use one part—for example, an arm in reaching—and hold back the rest of the body. This habit creates tension and compensation in other areas of the body, leading to chronic imbalance and misuse.

Gravity might be thought of as having a negative influence on the body. Indeed, when the body is out of balance, gravity pulls down on the parts that are out of line and reinforces their imbalance. Muscle tension develops as a result of trying to hold up the body, putting pressure on the joints. However when all parts are balanced within the

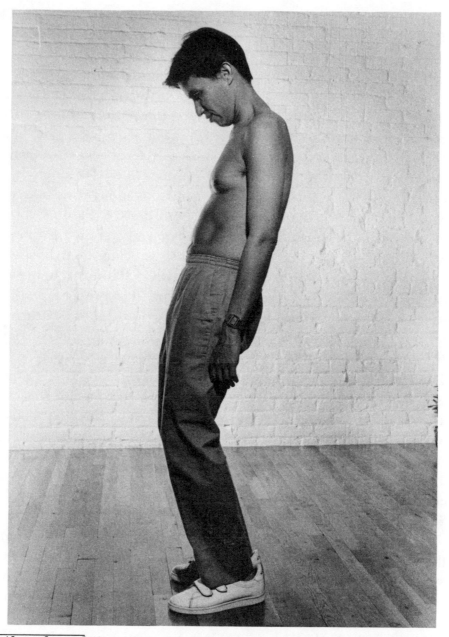

In Alexander technique, posture is important. Several points of poor posture are shown here: 1. Ankles give no support to legs and knees. 2. Knees give no support to waist. 3. Pelvis not extended properly. 4. Shoulders sag with no support from concave chest. 5. Neck is tilted too far down.

vertical arrangement, gravity actually supports the upward thrust. The body no longer has to hold on to itself, and the external, superficial muscles can release.

An underlying premise of the Alexander technique is that most people have lost their kinesthetic sense. The word *kinesthetic* is a combination of *kinetic* ("motion") and *esthetic* ("feeling"). The *kinesthetic sense,* therefore, can be defined as "a sense of motion or movement that is dependent on the ability to use neuromuscular feedback to determine what we are doing with our bodies." Through the interaction of the brain and muscles, we can coordinate conscious thought with action.

As we develop poor movement habits, our muscles become chronically shortened. The resulting imbalanced way of standing, sitting, or moving is perceived by our kinesthetic sense as being the correct way. If you habitually slouch in your favorite easy chair, eventually this pattern will feel familiar, right, and comfortable. The proper kinesthetic messages are no longer being received. It is the Alexander teacher's role to guide us into realizing where we have gone wrong, what the right patterns are, and how to sense and use them.

There are several theories about how we lost this kinesthetic awareness. Very often we may find ourselves moving in only a half-conscious state. We don't think about how we are bending to pick up a book or how we are combing our hair or sitting on a chair. This is not to suggest that we should monitor our every move; but as we become more aware of how we move, kinesthetic awareness becomes integrated into our every action.

Some people have proposed the genetic theory that, as bipeds, we have not completely integrated the upright posture. Although we may still be evolving into this posture, the fact remains that someone who has been functioning with a misused body (swayback or hunched shoulders, for example) can, after a series of Alexander lessons, return to balanced, well-aligned posture and body use.

It seems more likely that our tendency to misuse our bodies results mainly from the stresses of modern life. We have not changed much structurally, but we have adapted our bodies to a fast-changing environment and to specific styles in furniture, clothes, entertainment, and pace of life that are often not conducive to proper body use. Take the infant, for example, who moves with perfect balance. In coming into a sitting position, the child uses the body in a balanced way. If left to his or her own devices, the child will later stand and walk naturally. But this seldom happens, because parents who are eager to have the baby walk usually encourage the child to stand too soon either by putting it in a walker or supporting it by the hands and arms. This creates tension and imbalances, and already the child is on the way to chronic misuse of the body.

Emotional factors must also be considered. The position of the head pulled back and downward—an all too familiar sight—is akin to the action produced by the startle response or, as Alexander referred to it, the fear reflex. This and other emotions, if unreleased, become locked into our bodies, creating habitual tension.

The head, neck, and spine are the primary focus for the Alexander technique. The head, weighing from ten to fifteen pounds, can exert a considerable compression force on the spine. It is an important center for the body, housing the brain and major sense organs. If it is held in a balanced position, it will be supported by gravity and can lift off the spine. This allows the head to rotate freely on the neck and allows the spine to have full length and full range of motion. The spine, the core of the body, will have proper alignment and a free upward thrust, allowing the rest of the body to fall into place.

■ Techniques of the Alexander System

Practitioners of the Alexander technique are known as teachers, and those coming to receive the benefits are called students. This follows from Alexander's belief that proper use of the body is a learning experience. The Alexander teacher must know how to spot imbalances in the use of the body, no matter how minute, and be able to eliminate these imbalances in order to create a more aligned and integrated body structure.

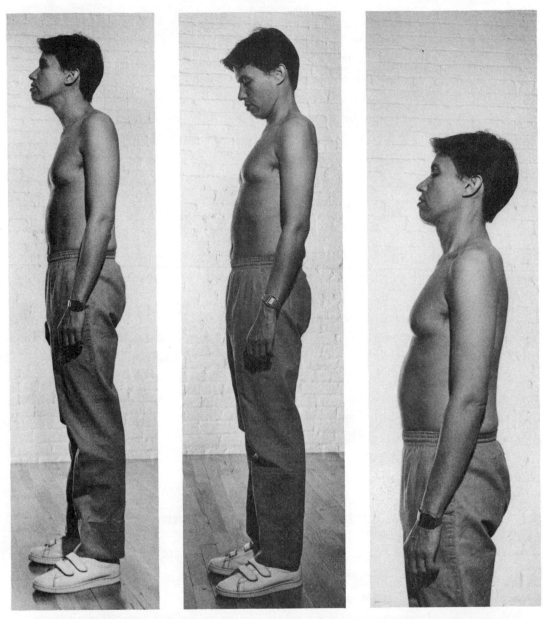

This is a good exercise for maintaining posture. Visualize a balloon with a string tied to it attached to the top of your head. The balloon slowly rises, pulling your head and neck in a slight extension.

Neck position may affect talking and singing. If the neck is hyperextended or tilted down too far, the air column is blocked and breathing is inhibited. Try singing in both positions. You will notice more fullness and control of your voice in the correct position.

Extension of the neck to improve voice and breathing.

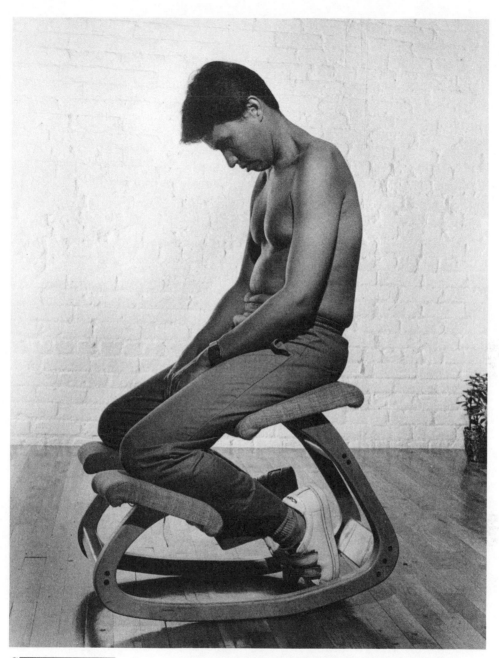

Sitting with the neck and back slumped may eventually lead to back pain. Back problems may be helped with the aid of specially designed chairs that relieve pressure from the spine and neck.

A session in Alexander technique usually takes from forty-five to sixty minutes. The teacher provides verbal instruction and physical guidance with the hands to coax misused muscles into better alignment. Concentration and a desire to change are required of the student, who must allow his or her body to respond to the teacher's instructions and guidance.

Chair and table work are used in most sessions, although some teachers may use only one or the other technique. Chair work involves teaching the student to use the body efficiently in moving from a sitting to a standing position and vice versa. The instruction involves the use of the major movement areas in the body: flexing at the hip and knee joints; alignment and direction of the head, neck, and spine; and balance of the shoulder girdle and arms.

Typical verbal instructions given by the teacher during this process are, "Let the neck be free to allow the head to move forward and up and to allow the spine to lengthen and the back to widen." A corollary instruction is to "allow the shoulders to widen and the knees to go forward." These are all "nondoing" words, which means that the student does not have to move or tense the body's muscles but can allow the suggestion to direct the deeper, more efficient muscles.

Table work is a more passive activity for the student. The teacher places his or her hands on various parts of the body and gently directs the student to lengthen and widen, thereby releasing tension and providing a new awareness of alignment and balance.

The organization of the session reinforces the main emphasis of the system: improving how we use our bodies in daily life. As the sessions progress, the teacher may incorporate other daily activities, such as teaching the student how to pick up objects properly, how to bend down, reach, push, walk, and run. The session is conducted in the student's regular clothes so that the "everydayness" of the activities is reinforced. It is through listening repeatedly to the teacher's instructions, feeling the guidance of the teacher's hands, and directing proper thoughts to the body that the student reeducates the kinesthetic sense and achieves proper use of the body.

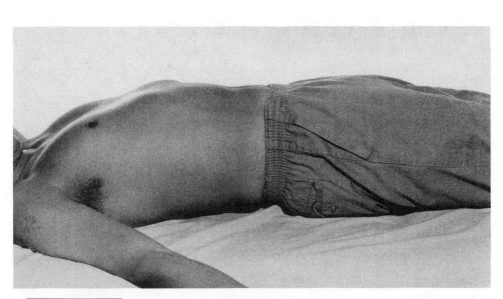

Back incorrectly arched while lying down, which creates tension under the buttocks and entire spine.

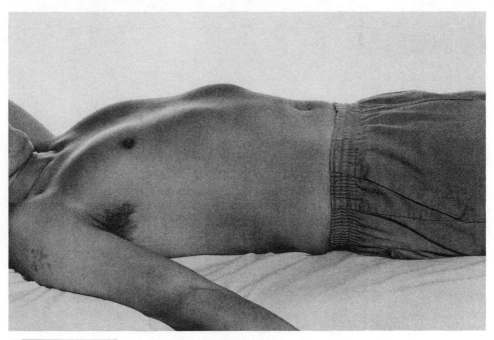

Back properly relaxed and flat, free of tension.

THE ALEXANDER TECHNIQUE   113

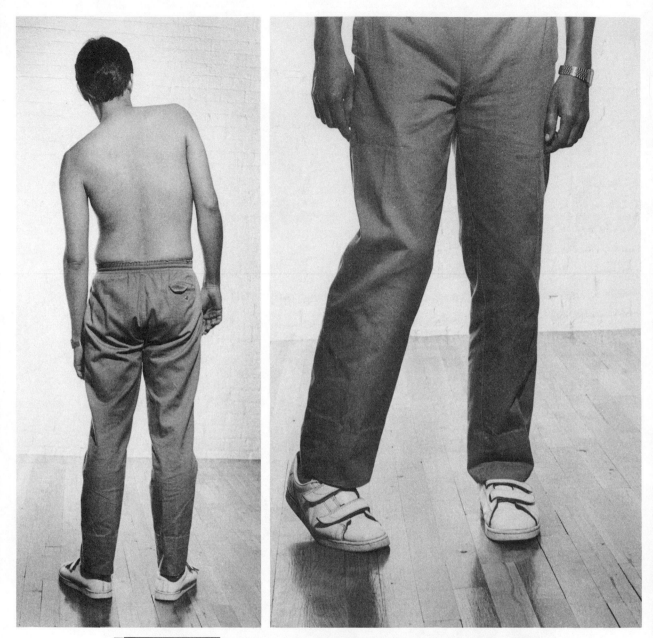

Tilted shoulders may have a negative effect on the neck. Drop your hands to your sides and look into the mirror to see if one hand is lower than the other. Then examine the shoulders to see if one shoulder is higher than the other. If so, straighten the shoulders by lifting the one that is lower.

Improper positioning of the feet. Feet are the base or foundation of the body, and just as the foundation of a house must be firm and planted securely, so should the feet. Proper standing can help maintain the entire body. Ankles that are turned or toes that are pointed excessively one way or the other may cause imbalances or leg problems.

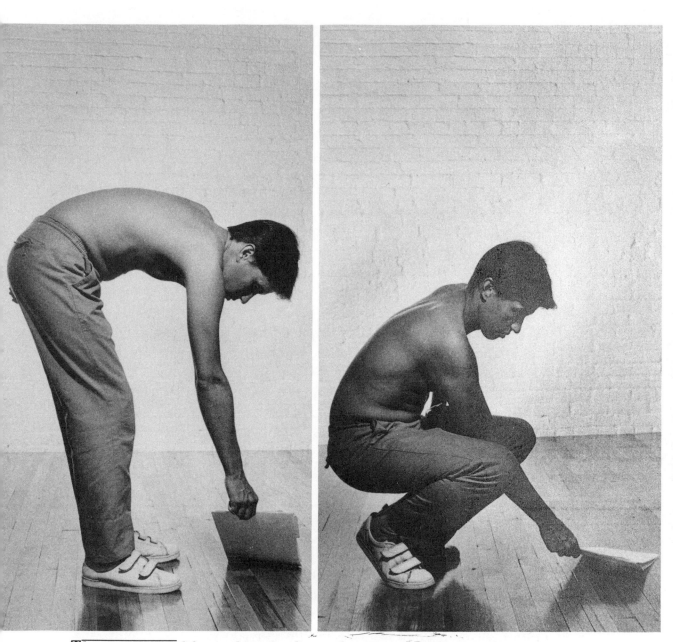

The wrong way to lift something. Bending at the waist puts undue pressure on the spine and may cause injury.

The correct way to lift. Bend the knees and stoop slowly. Avoid quick, jerky movements.

THE ALEXANDER TECHNIQUE   115

■ Training and Certification

Several schools in the United States and England offer certification in the Alexander technique. The major school in the United States is the American Center for the Alexander Technique (ACAT), located in New York City with a branch in San Francisco. The Carrington School and the McDonald School, founded by Walter Carrington and Patrick McDonald respectively, are the most well known Alexander schools in England. Other schools have branched off from these three and offer their own certification. Certified teachers who belong to the Society for Teachers of the Alexander Technique (STAT) can train students through their own certification programs. These students are then eligible to become members of STAT. The two major London schools and ACAT have similar standards and mutual recognition of certification.

Certification through ACAT requires three years of training at the school (the time requirement for the London schools is similar). Hands-on work constitutes 90 percent of the training. Other aspects involve the student's use of his or her own body (one private lesson a week is included), observation, and classes in anatomy. Requirements for admission include thirty private lessons with a certified teacher. Applicants also must possess a B.A. degree or equivalent and must demonstrate clarity in their own body use, although total body integration is not required at the time of admission.

■ Career Development

Most Alexander technique graduates go into private practice. Some work in schools, particularly with dance and drama departments, hospitals, performing arts organizations, and nursing homes. The possibilities for application are vast and include sports medicine and work in rehabilitative medicine. Since the technique is not well suited for group situations, one-on-one practices are the most common and effective.

■ How to Locate a Practitioner

In the United States, the ACAT serves as the central Alexander organization and publishes a directory of certified Alexander teachers. There are about 200 teachers certified through ACAT in the United States; the major concentrations are in New York and California. There are over 150 certified teachers in London and over 150 elsewhere in the world, including Israel, Europe, Canada, and Australia.

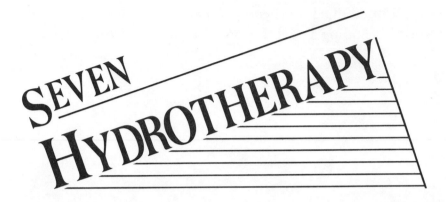

SEVEN HYDROTHERAPY

■ What Is Hydrotherapy?

Hydrotherapy is the scientific application of water in the treatment of imbalances or the application of water for cosmetic purposes. Hydrotherapy utilizes variations in the temperature of water, compresses, packs, and fomentations. These will be explained more fully later in this chapter.

Among the benefits of hydrotherapy are that it develops muscle tone; reduces inflammation or swelling, stimulates sluggish circulation; raises or lowers body temperature; stops bleeding, purifies the body by removing wastes; relieves congestion of blood, lymph, and other body fluids; unclogs the pores; and stimulates or sedates the nervous system.

Obviously one of the great advantages of hydrotherapy is its universal availability and low cost when done at home. We have only listed a few of the benefits of hydrotherapy techniques. Usually a series of treatments is needed. The best results are achieved when these are

118

used in conjunction with a program of internal cleansing and special diets of natural foods, fresh air, sunshine, and rest in a quiet retreat setting.

Hydrotherapy provides the greatest benefit when used in conjunction with skillful body massage. It can equalize circulation and produce a wonderful state of relaxation and peace of mind as well as provide release from physical and psychic stress.

■ Background and History of Hydrotherapy

Hydrotherapy goes back to ancient times and has been used by practically all cultures to maintain health and treat disease. For modern hydrotherapy techniques, however, we are indebted to the world-famous turn-of-the-century American physician John Harvey Kellogg. The pioneer of many home remedies, medical inventions, breakfast cereals, and exercises, Dr. Kellogg was the leading proponent of hydrotherapy up to World War II. Today we see hydrotherapy being conducted in many kinds of institutions, from European health spas to highly scientific medical centers in America.

The use of hydrotherapy became more popular when people began to turn away from the drug- and technology-oriented medical practices of the 1960s and 1970s. A leader in this field today is Richard A. Hansen, M.D., a prominent spokesman for the preventive health movement. He is a frequent lecturer and writer of the popular encyclopedia of home health care *Get Well at Home*.

Institutions throughout the country provide hydrotherapy in modern medical settings where expert diagnosis is available.

Internationally, hydrotherapy is practiced at centers at the Mount Akagi Institute in Japan; clinics in Belize in Central America; at the Hospital Yerba Buena in southern Mexico and also in Colombia, Venezuela, and Guatemala. Centers such as the Enton Hall Clinic in Surrey (just south of London) have been opened throughout Europe.

■ Principles and Philosophy of Hydrotherapy

Hydrotherapy induces balanced circulation, which can help heal every organ of the body, since good health depends upon good circulation. Because heat dilates the blood vessels and increases the blood flow, and cold does the opposite, these applications can decongest the head and chest, warm the body, reduce pelvic congestion, and speed healing in almost any infectious or inflammatory disease.

Everyone uses water in some form daily, whether it's soaking tired feet, taking a long hot shower, or just having a refreshing glass of cool water on a hot summer day. Human beings can live much longer without food than without water. Water distributes nutrients to all the cells of the body, carries out toxins, and comprises two-thirds of the body's tissues. For therapeutic effects as an adjunct to massage, water can be used hot or cold, either as a liquid, a solid (ice), or a gas (steam). When combined wih herbs and other agents, its therapeutic effects are enhanced. With massage or bodywork, water helps loosen and relax muscles.

■ Hydrotherapy Techniques

Hydrotherapy may involve the use of a massage or treatment table, where the subject lies relaxed—prone or supine—with hot packs applied to the feet, the spine, or other affected parts of the body. General aches and pains, as well as stress and tension, are rapidly reduced by the use of appropriate hydrotherapy. Techniques are described in a number of books, such as *Get Well at Home,* by Dr. Hansen (see Resources section). Full-body whirlpool, sitz bath, Turkish and Russian steam baths are also used as adjuncts to the approaches of hydrotherapy. Often treatments end with cold mitten friction or a contrast spray. This tones the body and is more stimulating than any cup of coffee or even a cold plunge in the ocean!

The techniques of massage (usually the Swedish variety) that follow these applications include the following four general movements: First, there is *effleurage* or stroking movements, in which the skillful hands of the therapist empty the veins toward the heart and soothe and relax the skin and underlying muscles. The next step is kneading, sometimes called *petrissage,* which involves the further stimulation of muscles, particularly those under tension or in spasm. The percussion effect, *tapotement,* involves the further stimulation of muscles, taking care to avoid tender or painful areas that may react adversely. *Vibration* is another common form of massage, either done manually or with an appropriate electrical device. Systematically, the extremities are treated one at a time, followed by the back and finally the trunk. Specialized massage applications on the face and head produce dramatic effects in release of tension and headache.

The lubricants used are oil (such as bath oil, aromatic compounds, or pine-scented oil) or an appropriate cream. The treatment rooms are quiet and warm, and the therapist's attitude must always be sensitive to the needs of each patient as the treatment progresses.

Some specific hydrotherapy techniques include:

- *Alternating baths*   The use of hot water in a first bath and cold water in a following bath. The hot water first dilates the blood vessels, which improves the circulation and helps remove waste products from the area. Next, the cold water greatly increases blood flow to that area. Repeat this three times, as follows: First, three minutes in hot water. Next, cold water for three minutes, and so on. (This procedure may be done in the shower.) It can also be used with the Water-Pik massage shower, which produces pulsating streams of water that relieve tired or aching muscles. Arthritis responds very well to the alternating baths treatment.
- *Colonic irrigation*   Usually a licensed nurse or a certified colon therapist will be able to offer these services. It is best to consult with your physician before obtaining a colonic irrigation. However, the procedure is generally known to be safe and painless. Colonic irrigation has become a popular way of

cleansing the internal system, providing more energy and relief from digestive problems such as diarrhea or constipation. It can help rejuvenate the entire system over a series of sessions if it is combined with a healthful, cleansing diet, which aids in detoxifying the entire body.

The purpose of colonic irrigation is to wash out the colon. Unlike an enema, the colonic will also wash the wall of the intestines.

Colonics involve the injection into the colon of a large amount of water or water and herbs that fill the colon and totally flush and clean it out. Two primary methods are used: (a) The one-tube method, whereby the colon is filled to capacity through a single tube and the liquid runs out through the same tube; and (b) the two-tube method, where separate tubes are used for inflow and outflow.

- *Fomentations*   These are useful to relieve congestion in the chest, colds, and respiratory imbalances such as bronchitis and flu. They also relieve pain in neuralgia, arthritis, and other inflammation. A fomentation is the application of moist heat to the body's skin. Use a cloth that contains 50 percent wool (to retain heat) and 50 percent cotton (to retain moisture).

To make a fomentation, fold your cloth into manageable size, boil a pot of water, boil the folded cloth in the pot of water, then remove, cool until handleable, and apply it to the area you wish to stimulate. Leave it there for three to five minutes. Repeat this two more times. When the fomentation has been removed, take a clean cotton washcloth and rub the skin with cold water. To finish, dry the skin thoroughly.

- *Compresses*   A compress prevents the circulation of air and allows heat to accumulate around the affected area. It may be used to cover the knee, wrist, or any area needing this type of application.

To make a compress, use a clean strip of cotton cloth to wrap the area at least twice. If you are using a hot compress, soak it in boiling water; wring the water out and cover the area. Be sure it is not so hot that it causes damage to the skin surface but is hot enough to be effective. If a cold compress is used, soak it in cold water and follow the same procedure. After wrapping it around the treatment area, pin or clip it so that it remains intact.

To make a compress for sore throat or laryngitis, use a cotton cloth large enough to cover the entire throat area. Add a drop of oil of pepperment to the cloth while immersed in warm water. Wrap the compress around throat and cover with the same size material made of heavy cotton or flannel. Clip or pin with safety pins and leave on overnight. When removing, wash the throat with a loofah sponge or heavy cotton washcloth.

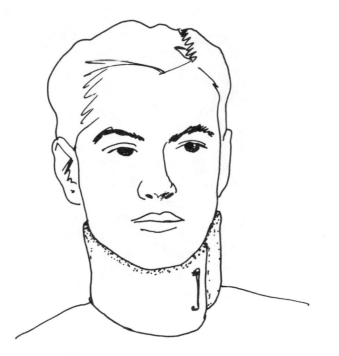

Heat compress.

■ *Ice packs* Can be used to reduce soreness or swelling. If capillaries or arteries are injured, ice packs will prevent further damage and prevent swelling. (Remember, ice cold water contracts blood vessels and inhibits the flow of circulation, allowing the area time to heal itself.) Cold compresses also help allay pain and discomfort, creating a mild anesthetic effect.

Using a foot bath or bathtub, immerse the body part in water as cold as you can stand it. Keep it there for at least fifteen minutes and repeat every two hours until you have received five treatments. An ice pack may be more convenient in some situations. If you do not have one available, put ice cubes in a clean cotton towel and apply directly to the skin.

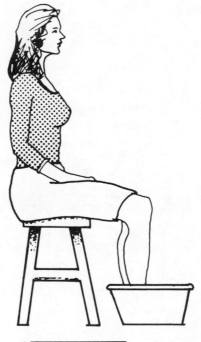

Cold foot bath.

- *Steam inhalation* Inhalation of steam will help clear the sinuses, open blocked bronchial tubes, increase respiration, and clean toxins from the skin while it helps with difficult breathing. It relieves the feeling of stiffness. By keeping the pores open and clean, steam helps the skin look better and maintain its natural glow. Inside the home or office, dry air may exist due to heat, air conditioners, or poor air quality. Vaporizers are available, which heat water and generate steam. When using a vaporizer, you may wish to add a small quantity of herbs such as peppermint or chamomile to increase the effectiveness.

   For a vaporizing effect, use either a vaporizer by Clairol or humidifier by Kaz for a cool mist. Both increase moisture in the environment.

   For an old-fashioned steam facial that cleans skin and reduces blemishes and pimples, boil 3 cups of water, remove pot from stove, pour water into large bowl, add 2 cupfuls of AUNU Herbal Sauna, if desired. Place a towel over your head, creating a tent, and allow steam to penetrate skin. Lightly massage facial area. The AUNU health and beauty products are a total approach to natural beauty. Information may be obtained from: AUNU, Ansonia Station #1206, New York, NY 10023 (203-838-9940).

- *Hot tubs and whirlpools* Used in some countries for years, these are now readily available and easy to maintain. They may be used wherever space and plumbing permit.

- *Flotation or isolation tanks* A unique way to relax the total body and relieve the muscles of excess tension. Upon relaxing in a solution of water and epsom salts, the body reaches a state known as zero gravity. It is at zero gravity that no undue force or gravitational pull is applied on the body. The body floats in a serene, quiet, and peaceful atmosphere. Usually a session will last for one hour.

   Results vary. Testimonies from people who have had flo-

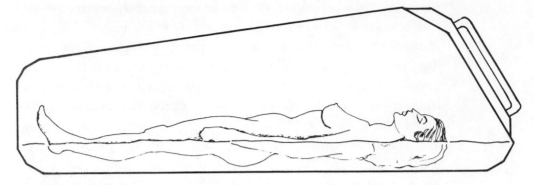

Flotation tank.

tation sessions reveal they have experienced an increase in assertive energy, feelings of calmness, clarity of mind, and reduction of pain associated with sore or aching muscles.

■ *Swimming*   This is the ultimate exercise! During swimming, nature takes over, providing both fun and relaxation. While swimming builds strong muscle tone, it provides a wonderful technique of self-massage. Swimming offers the following benefits:

It builds and strengthens muscles, especially in legs, chest, and arms.
It increases respiration for better breathing.
It improves circulation and blood flow.
It massages muscles for relief of aches and pains.
It provides relaxation.

If you are using a pool, be sure to wear goggles for eye protection. Also use a swimming cap, as pool chemicals are very damaging to the hair. Take safety precautions, and if you're not an excellent swimmer, be sure to swim only in protected areas, especially in natural surroundings.

■ Training and Certification

Practitioners of hydrotherapy become expert through many years of practice in institutions that have developed over the past forty years in America. The well-known Wildwood Sanitarium and Hospital in Wildwood, Georgia, is the parent institution, with its training seminars in nursing arts, its fellowships for physicians and other medical professionals, and its special training programs in nutrition, hydrotherapy, and massage. The latter courses are of six to twelve months in length, with a great deal of hands-on experience and a very moderate tuition charge.

■ Career Opportunities

The opportunities for practitioners of hydrotherapy are abundant in clinics opening in major cities of North America and Europe as well as the third world nations.

EIGHT
ESTHETIC MASSAGE

Since days of old, beauty has been one of the most sought after treasures by both women and men. Why not be beautiful? There is an old saying that beauty is only skin deep. Beauty is truly a reflection that begins inside. The esthetic massage program incorporates elements that help create a healthier state inside the body that results in a more beautiful appearance. Esthetic massage is composed of massage, hydrotherapy, exercise, nutrition, and positive visualization.

Centuries ago massage was used as a method of promoting facial beauty. Women bathed their faces in the Nile or the Euphrates, experiencing their healthy and rich waters. Later on, exercises, along with the use of certain natural plants or exotic herbs, were combined to aid in this quest. History informs us that hydrotherapy, facial massage, exercise, and the other components of esthetic massage have long been used not only in the Middle East but also in the Orient and throughout South America. Today we know much more about the human body, including the muscles, tissues, and bones, and the structure of the face and the needs of the skin.

Esthetic massage is a metamorphosis of many effective techniques. Although there are few certified practitioners of this technique, it is extremely effective and useful. Aspects of it are designed as self-help.

Esthetic massage is not only designed for face and skin but also for every part of the body—hands, feet, hair, and legs. The system includes nutritional components that help regenerate and preserve the body's health, rather than degenerate and devitaminize the body. Dietary recommendations include vitamins, minerals, herbs, and special supplements, along with monitoring the intake of white sugar, white flour, salt, and other foods. Each person's biochemical makeup is different. Nutritional needs vary from one person to another. Therefore, it is necessary to look at each person's living habits. There are, however, certain general nutritional practices that have been accepted as being universally helpful. Once these practices, following, are incorporated, a person's nutritional habits are increased in quality by 50 percent.

- Balance the intake of vitamins, minerals, carbohydrates, and proteins.
- Never eat when upset.
- Avoid eating heavy meals before going to bed.
- Eat more fruit and fresh vegetables and less fat and red meat.
- Drink fresh juices, which provide valuable life sustaining enzymes.
- Be sure you consume the required daily amounts of nutrients, via food or supplements.
- Only eat what your system needs. Excess food will develop into fat or waste.
- Consume citrus fruits regularly, because they cleanse the system and eliminate toxins from the body.

The process of the ultimate facial renewal begins with a look at the special needs of each individual. Since the face and skin respond to stimuli, the application of therapeutic elements such as water, oils, heat, and cold and the use of specially designed movements definitely have the power to make changes in the appearance.

Some of the benefits of facial rejuvenation are to:

- increase circulation
- activate cellular tissues below the skin surface
- increase tone of muscles and tissues
- reduce unwanted surface lines and wrinkles
- open clogged pores for better circulation
- bring nutrients to skin surface
- tighten sagging skin
- dilate, or open, blood vessels, improving circulation and relieving congestion
- act as a cleanser, helping eliminate wastes and toxins
- help delay atrophy of the muscles
- improve general circulation and bring nutrients to muscles
- encourage retention of nitrogen, phosphorus, and sulphur, necessary for repairing the tissues

You will find that the system of esthetic massage outlined here is unique. After realizing the positive benefits received by many clients who sought a safe and effective technique for beautifying the face and skin, I found the need to offer this system in an easy-to-follow method. Combining the best from massage techniques, hydrotherapy, nutrition, and exercise, the results are astounding. In some cases, the final result has lifted years from the appearance of the body. In the words of one recipient, it brings an apparent glow to the entire body. Another described it as finding the fountain of youth. Still another description was, "My entire body feels rejuvenated."

There are no medical claims to this system. It simply works. The concept is to approach the face with a caring, gentle attitude, one that revolves around the needs of the client. Firming the muscle tone and adding elasticity to the skin at the same time is the first goal. Since the musculature of the face determines the effect of unwanted lines and furrows in the face, it is important to manipulate the muscles, following

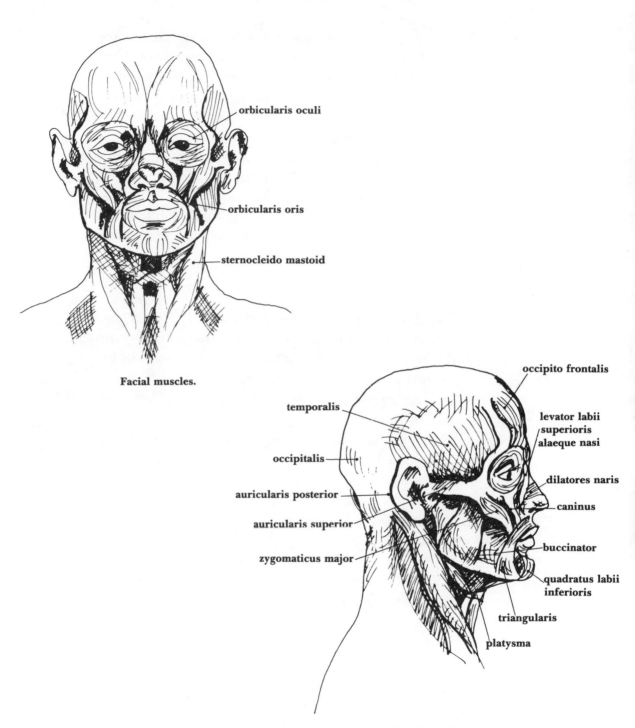

orbicularis oculi

orbicularis oris

sternocleido mastoid

Facial muscles.

occipito frontalis

temporalis

levator labii
superioris
alaeque nasi

occipitalis

dilatores naris

auricularis posterior

caninus

auricularis superior

zygomaticus major

buccinator

quadratus labii
inferioris

triangularis

platysma

Facial muscles.

the diagram of the anatomy. On the other hand, there are several effective techniques that bypass the anatomy and involve the energy system of the body. These may include pressure points, energy pathways, and emotional attitudes. Happiness, joy, and self-confidence lead to a glowing, vibrant complexion, while sadness, jealousy, and displeasure may lead to many skin conditions. It is important to realize the connection of body, mind, and emotions. This chapter could be titled, Make Yourself Young and Beautiful, as certainly the approach extends far beyond simple facial massage.

Literally, this new and exciting massage method offers you beauty at your fingertips. It will give you instructions on techniques you can perform on yourself, at any time.

Some basic facts about your skin:

- The skin is the largest organ of the body.
- It acts as a mirror for internal imbalances and disorders.
- It acts as a protective layer for the internal organs by keeping out dirt and other particles.
- It is composed of nerves, tissues, and muscle; hair follicles and oil glands.
- The layers include the outer layer, known as the epidermis, the middle layer, or the dermis, and the subcutaneous middle layer. The middle layer contains a structural protein known as collagen. Collagen gives skin elasticity, allowing it to stretch. Collagen breaks down with age, causing the skin to stretch and sag.
- It helps regulate body temperature.
- It serves as a vehicle for nutrients to enter the body.
- It has nerve sensors that respond to hot and cold.
- It helps regulate blood pressure.
- An important function is the elimination of waste materials and the release of toxins from the body.
- It also breathes, absorbing oxygen and expelling carbon dioxide.

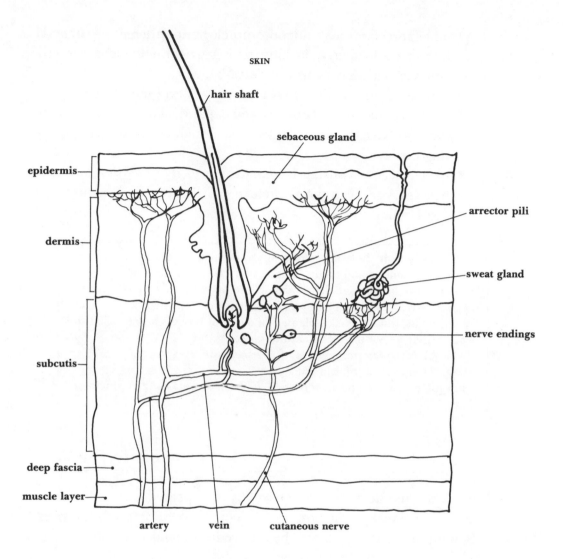

SKIN

hair shaft

sebaceous gland

epidermis

dermis

arrector pili

sweat gland

subcutis

nerve endings

deep fascia

muscle layer

artery vein cutaneous nerve

- The tissues around the eyes are soft and thin. Be supercareful when massaging around this delicate area.
- Oily skin occurs when the oil glands are too active, thus producing an overabundance of oil. Also humidity, environment, dry or moist air, and nutritional factors will have an effect on this.

- The pores of oily skin become clogged, preventing it from breathing properly, locking toxins in the skin and thereby causing blackheads and pimples.
- The skin is nourished by blood vessels and capillaries.
- Because it is able to contract and expand, skin allows the body parts to have freedom of movement, such as stretching, reaching, etc.
- Skin cells are constantly renewing and dying. Therefore it is necessary to keep the skin clean to rid the body constantly of dead cells.

> To supplement the esthetic massage approach, a leading chemist has developed a unique and natural line of skin care products whose purpose is to offer the finest ingredients available to accompany a facial massage regimen. AUNU includes moisture treatments, refining masks, toners, eye cream, revitalizing massage oil, and lotion. It also offers a line of natural brushes that follow the face's natural contours.
>
> The AUNU program consists of five basic steps: cleansing, steaming, refining, toning, and moisturizing.
>
> For information on how to order AUNU esthetic massage products, see page 155.

■ Problems in the Face

Some lines in the face are caused by a repeated action, such as smiling. Also, the expression of certain emotions can stretch the muscles. Some basic conditions can be relieved by facial massage.

- Wrinkles can occur when the skin loses its elasticity or can be a result of worry and excessive thinking, which may leave lines in the forehead. They can also be a result of the tissues and muscles shrinking. Facial skin begins to sag and fold. When deep wrinkles form, the skin fibers begin to break and the skin also begins to thin.

- Crow's feet are action lines caused by stretching of the skin over the eye area. They may show several layers of wrinkles and may also be caused by squinting.
- Sagging cheeks are collapsed upper cheek muscles.
- Horizontal lines in the forehead may be caused by excessive thinking.
- Vertical lines in the forehead may be caused by excessive worry.
- Scowl lines are formed by continually pulling the brows together.
- Sagging eyebrows are collapsed muscles in the upper eyelids.
- A line in the bridge of the nose is an action line from knotting the brow.
- Tight jaw or pain in the sides of the face is called TMJ (temperomandibular joint). Often tension is held in this area and may cause discomfort or even tight skin.
- Discoloration under the eyes may be caused by a kidney imbalance or drinking too many liquids.
- Acne, blackheads, and pimples may be a result of too much oil being released from the subcutaneous or oil glands. They may also be caused by emotional upset, anger, or fear or they may be the result of poor circulation or clogged pores.

■ Special Treatments for Facial Problems

It is important to remember that some conditions in the face are the result of habitual expressions. Ultimately these expressions leave a furrow or groove in the skin, which can be called a wrinkle.

Therefore the first and probably most important way to prevent facial problems is to stop making the particular expression. It can be from smiling, frowning, squinting, and so on.

To prevent *crow's feet,* open the eyes wide. Eye creams may help restore balance to the delicate tissue of the eye area. Warm facial packs can be made from cotton or muslin cloth. Apply on the eye area until the cloth becomes cool.

A good remedy for *sagging cheeks* is inverted posture. Use a slant board or some other furniture that will allow you to invert the head so that it is lower than the remainder of the body. Try this position at least fifteen minutes a day. The importance of gravity reversal is that it speeds the movement of blood back to your heart and head. Thus you take pressure away from potential varicose veins in legs and liven your facial tone in the process. A must for everyone, sagging cheeks or not!

To counteract *horizontal lines in the forehead,* first raise the eyebrows and the eye as if you were attempting to look at the top of your head. Hold for about ten seconds. This prepares the muscle. Next, begin with the forehead and rub the forehead back to the base of the neck. Use the fingertips to pull the skin back and to stroke the muscle back.

Use small, short strokes on the base of the neck. As you begin just under the scalp, work down toward the back. As you finish with one spot, move to the next spot on the neck, moving one-half inch each time.

Deep furrows between the eyes may be caused by *scowling.* Since these may be action lines, it is best to become aware of and avoid pulling the brows together. Excessive worrying or overconcern can lead to the habit of squeezing or pulling the brows together. A technique for breaking this habit is as follows:

Look in the mirror. Study the center of the forehead, between the eyes. Now pull the brows together, close your eyes, and focus your mind on this area. While you are still holding, remember what it feels like. Release the tension and repeat this.

The next time you have a problem or even a small concern, remember to examine this area. If you are holding tension in the area, focus on it and release the tension. Repeat techniques for exercises for horizontal lines. Next place both hands in the center of the forehead and stroke them out toward the ears, just as if you were rubbing away the scowl lines.

While nutritional deficiencies or water imbalances can cause *puffiness under the eyes*, lack of fresh air and rest can also be factors. Use ice or cold water packs (see p. 124).

■ Facial Exercises

Exercise can help prevent the deep lines or wrinkles caused by facial tension. Recommended times are morning or just before bed. Facial exercises, overall, stimulate circulation in the face, and may even nourish skin cells.

Approach each exercise in a relaxed manner, isolating each part as you exercise it.

Gradually inhale at the start of a particular position, and exhale when releasing the position. The quality of each is far more important than how many or how fast you perform each.

- Lion pose—rejuvenates the entire face. Take a deep breath and hold for about ten seconds. Exhale while counting to 15, letting the breath go slowly. Remember to inhale through your nose and exhale through your mouth.
- Pucker your lips as though you were giving someone a great big kiss. Make the movement to pucker, quick, and hold it for about ten seconds. Repeat this 3 times.
- Open the mouth wide as you say "aaahh." Hold for about ten seconds. Close the mouth and repeat again 2 more times.
- Squeeze the teeth inside the mouth with the lips closed. Bite down on the back of the mouth. Hold for about ten seconds. Repeat 3 times.

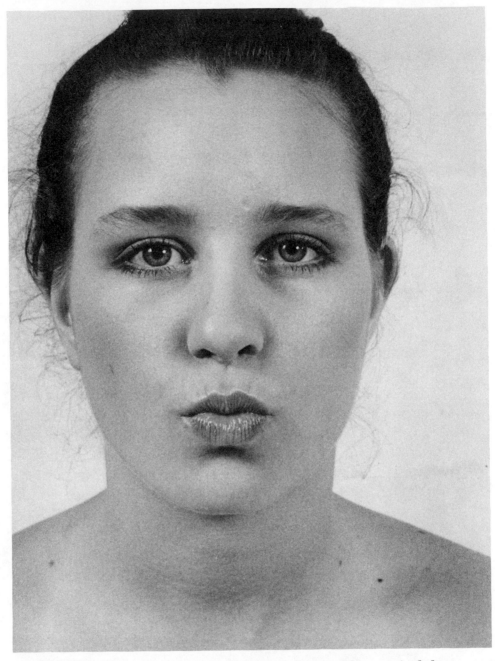

Pucker the lips and hold for ten seconds. Repeat 3 times. This exercise helps prevent smile lines.

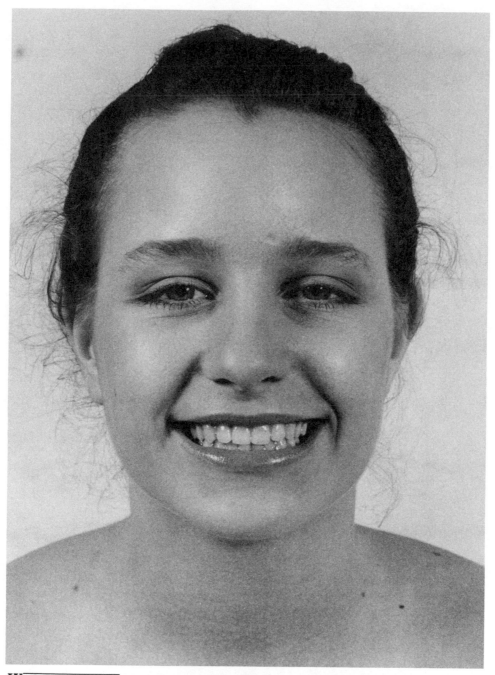

With teeth clenched lightly, spread your lips, as in smiling.

■ The Importance of Muscles in Maintaining Your Beauty

Muscles are a type of tissue composed of fibers and cells that give support and movement to an organ or an entire part of the body. The facial muscles can contract or expand as we smile, frown, chew, or speak. They add elasticity to the skin, making it supple and flexible. Where the skin begins to sag, perhaps a muscle is in a state of atrophy or deterioration. Proper tone can prevent this sagging. Through the voluntary will of our thought processes and isometric exercises, we can change the appearance of the face or give it better tone.

Even a face-lift can be facilitated by exercises and massage techniques that alter the present form of the muscles by returning their proper tone and elasticity. Also, by increasing the strength and mass of a muscle, it is possible to restore a glowing appearance to the face. This can be achieved through nutrients and improvement in the all-important circulation.

Good muscle tone will also help the functioning of eating, talking, vision, singing, and breathing. Deterioration of a muscle in the face can be a result of lack of nourishment, underuse, or aging.

■ Preparing for Facial Massage

1. Calm your mind.
2. Focus on the desired result.
3. Rub your hands together.

Rubbing the hands together brings warmth to them and removes any excess tension. The most important step in the session may very well be the beginning. In the beginning of the session, you set the tone for the application of touch. If you touch the face with tense and tight hands, you will most certainly transfer this tension to your face. So relax the hands before you touch.

Exercises that can help prepare the hands:

- Rotate the wrists by moving them in small circles, first clockwise 10 times, then counterclockwise 10 times.
- Rotate the fingers, beginning with the thumb and then each finger consecutively. Rotate in each direction 10 times.
- Shake the hands to remove excess tension.
- Now rub the hands together again until you feel the heat begin to pulsate in the palms of your hands.

■ Preparing the Environment

You may find the following items helpful in preparing for your session:

- small cotton towel
- massage oil
- massage table or chair with head rest
- soft facial tissues
- relaxing music
- soft light (perhaps green or blue, known for their relaxing effect)
- mirror (if you are doing facial self-massage)

The client should inhale very slowly, counting to 10. Then exhale through the mouth, counting to 15. Repeat this 2 more times. Place your hands about 3 inches away from the chin on the front of the face up to the scalp, feeling for a gentle pulsation along a line of total facial energy.

As your client relaxes, give the face a chance to relax. You may ask your client to do this special beauty visualization: "Relax your mind and just let all your thoughts and all outside interferences fall from your mind. While you are doing this, visualize yourself inside your mind; that is, see yourself as though you were in a field of pink carnations. Visualize the color of pink and see total pink reflect from the field of carnations over your entire face. For better visualization, see your face as it becomes penetrated by a large ray of pink sunshine. The rays are emitted from the sunshine and cover your entire face. Bathe your face in the color pink and feel the color pink bring new beauty to you."

Also very important in the esthetic massage system is the concept of seeing your face the way you want it to be. The beauty of your skin can be an asset to every part of your life. Not only is the beauty beneficial in your personal and social life, but a more beautiful, successful, vibrant-looking person certainly has more and greater opportunities in the world for success. Looking and feeling good both have their positive effects. The purpose of esthetic massage is to bring a better skin tone and a more vibrant feeling to the entire body—especially, in this case, to the face and to the skin.

There is a feeling and a look of youthfulness as esthetic massage actually works to create and help enforce better circulation. Through firmness of muscles and toning of the muscles or even the release of a tight muscle, the natural appearance is enhanced as a glow rises to the surface of the skin.

When touching the face, which we know is a sensitive area, it is best to start with less pressure and gradually apply a bit more pressure.

For smile lines, action lines, or any place where deep furrows or wrinkles exist, apply pressure longer than usual. Remember to approach with tension-free, relaxed hands. Many of us have a tremendous amount of tension in our hands, and it is best to free this tension before attempting any type of massage or self-massage. Also, always begin by taking a long, deep breath. These two elements are more important than learning all the techniques. Esthetic massage is based on the quality of touch rather than the quantity of touch or the number of techniques involved. If the quality of touch is superior and the right movements are made, the system is designed to give immediate and visible results. Usually after one session, you will notice and feel results. Later, after several sessions or self-sessions, you will notice long-lasting results. Based on a combination of anatomy, physiology, and energy pathways, esthetic massage takes into consideration the structure and functions of muscles, tissues, energy centers, and attitudes.

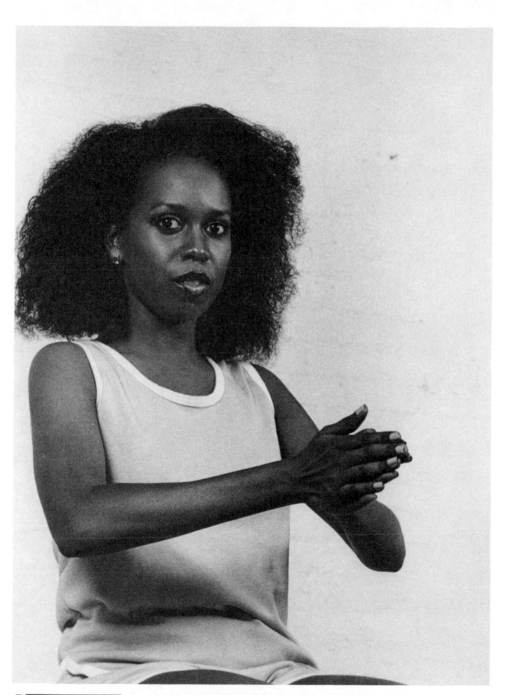

Preparing the hands. Rub them lightly until you feel a slight heat before beginning.

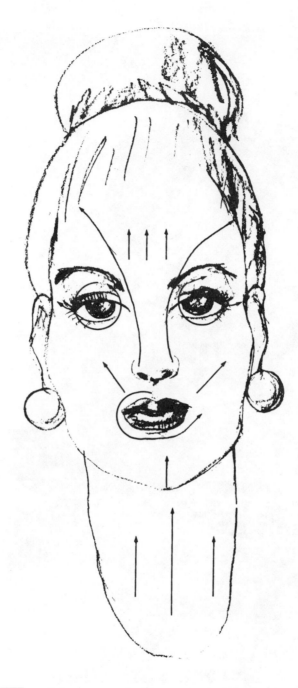

Follow the direction of these arrows when massaging the face or applying makeup.

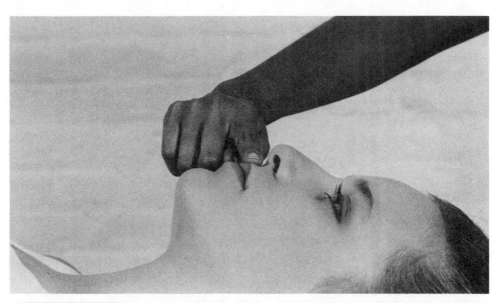

Press lightly under nose. This helps relieve tightness in jaw and teeth.

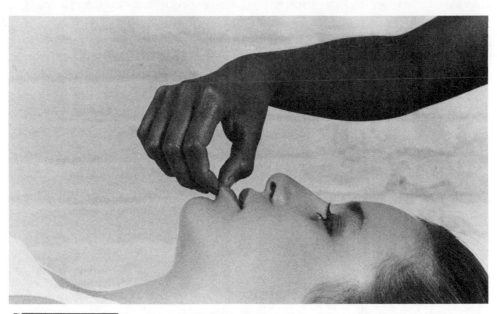

Gently lift upper lip and pull lightly, then squeeze along the lip line. Repeat to bottom lip. This esthetic massage technique increases circulation to the lips to give them a glossy, healthy look.

When you hold on to any negative feelings, whether it be sadness, jealousy, resentment, or hatred, you will cause your facial muscles to atrophy to a great degree. There will be less of an apparent glow on your face. Be careful; it shows! On the other hand, when you are generally happy and tend to be forgiving, understanding, and unselfish, your face will have a more positive and healthy aura.

Emotions and attitudes do play an important role in the structure and beauty of our faces, but it is also important to rest and get plenty of oxygen for vital, beautiful, glowing skin. Also, some cleansing brushes, such as AUNU's Maso brush and the Accu brush, are helpful in stimulating skin tissue, bringing fresh tone and circulation to the surface.

Hydrotherapy, the application of water, has been included here because of its practical and effective methods for increasing and firming skin tone. Saunas, whirlpool baths, steam rooms, compresses, and packs are all recommended components of the esthetic massage system.

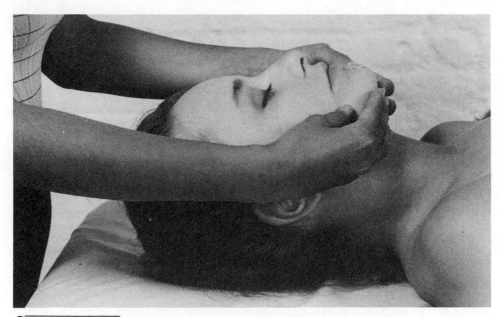

Stroking the neck. Begin at the breast bone and stroke up to chin.

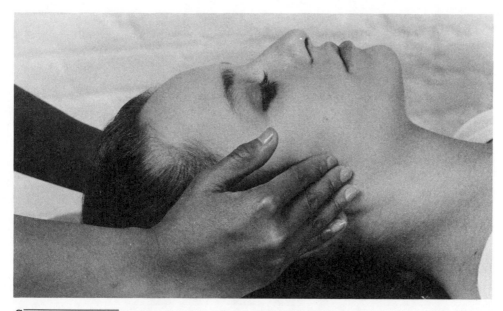

Stroking entire face. Begin at the base of the chin, stroke up across the ear, and back toward the scalp.

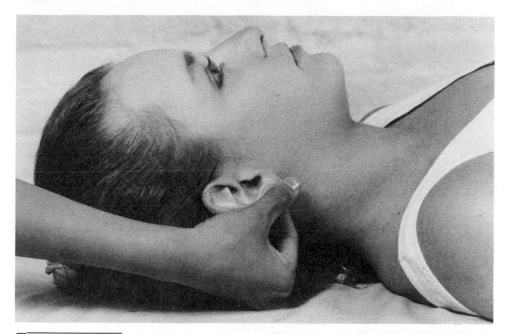

The ear is the connection point for several facial muscles. Stroking the ears helps relieve tightness in the face. Begin with the top and move toward the earlobe.

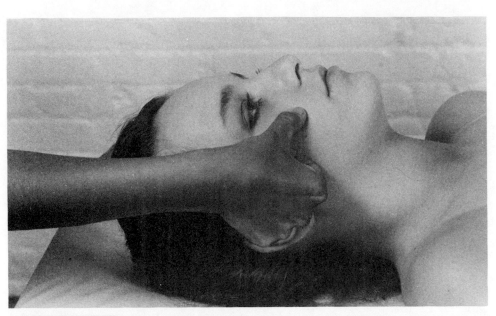

Apply slight pressure to a point in the center of the side of your face directly in line with your eye when looking straight ahead.

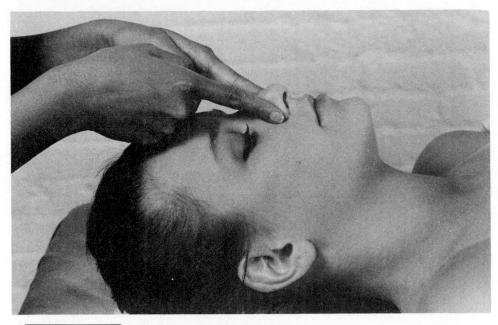

Apply slight pressure to the side of each nostril.

148   MASSAGE TECHNIQUES

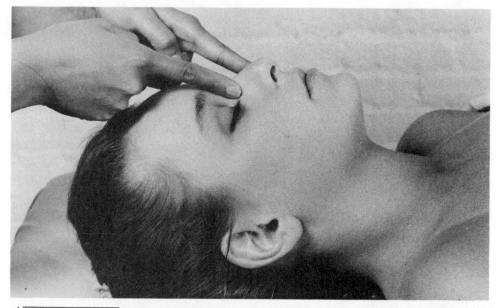

Apply slight pressure to the sides of the nose, then stroke the skin up toward the forehead.

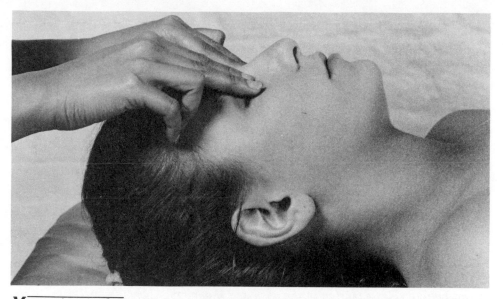

Massaging tired eyes. With the patient's eyes closed, place the palms of the fingertips over each eye. Rotate gently in clockwise circles. Then repeat with counterclockwise circles. Finally, apply gentle pressure to each eye.

ESTHETIC MASSAGE   149

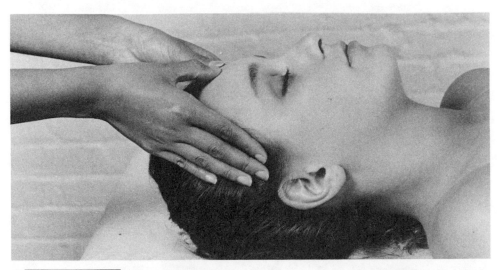

Excessive worrying or squinting may cause lines in the forehead. Relaxation techniques may help clear your mind. Using fingertips, firmly stroke the entire forehead up toward the scalp.

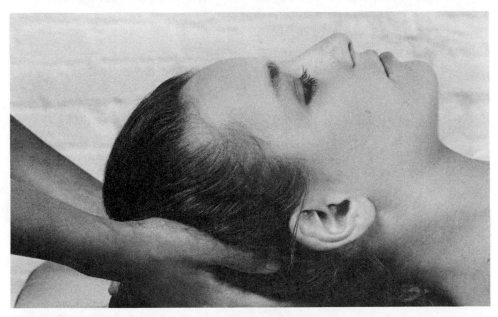

Head hold to release tension in the neck and shoulders. Place the fingertips on the base of the scalp, where the bone ends, and apply pressure. Hold for at least one minute. Focus on the breathing of the patient and ask the person to breathe slowly and to relax.

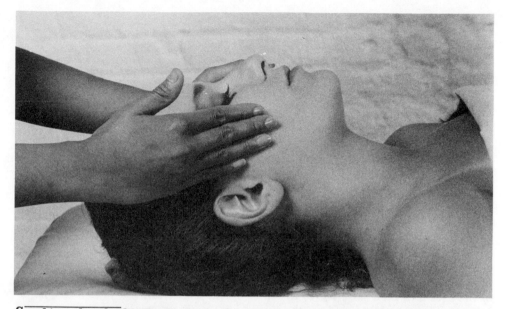

Stroking the cheeks. Begin at the base of the chin on both sides and stroke up toward the ear with long, firm strokes of the fingertips. This is soothing to the skin surface while stimulating circulation in this area.

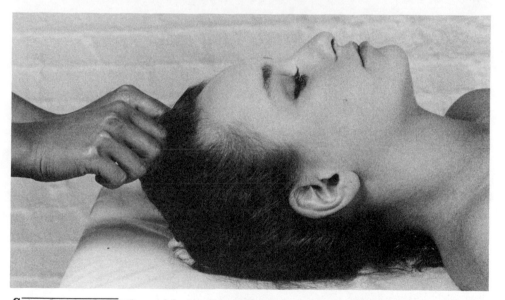

Stimulating the scalp and hair. Grasp the hair between the fingertips and lightly pull as you lean back.

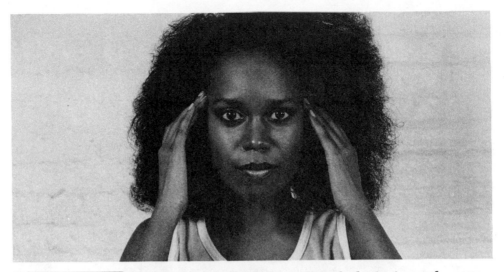

*R*ubbing the temples. *Rotate your fingertips in small circles beginning at the corners of the eyes and then move out to the sides of the face. Next, use your index finger to stroke in a straight line from the corner of the eye out toward the ear.*

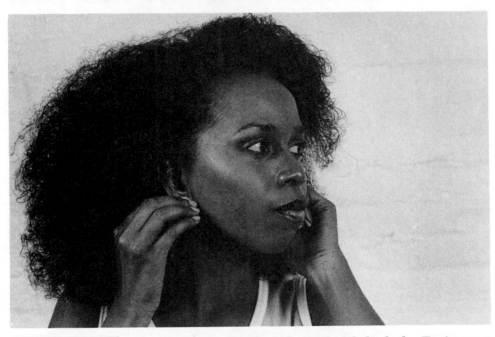

*S*troking the earlobe. *The earlobe is the coolest part of the body. To increase circulation, use short, firm strokes and stroke from top of ear to earlobe.*

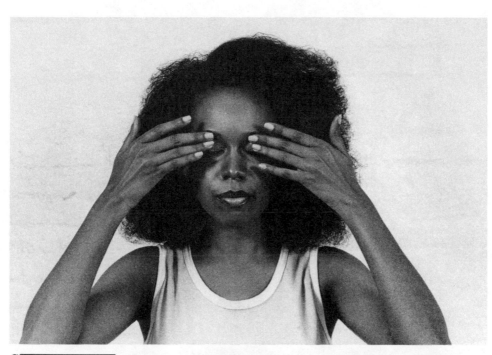

Self-massage for beautiful eyes. Apply gentle pressure by leaning your face into your fingertips. Hold for seven seconds. Repeat 3 times. Then rotate fingers in small, then large circles. Rotate in each direction.

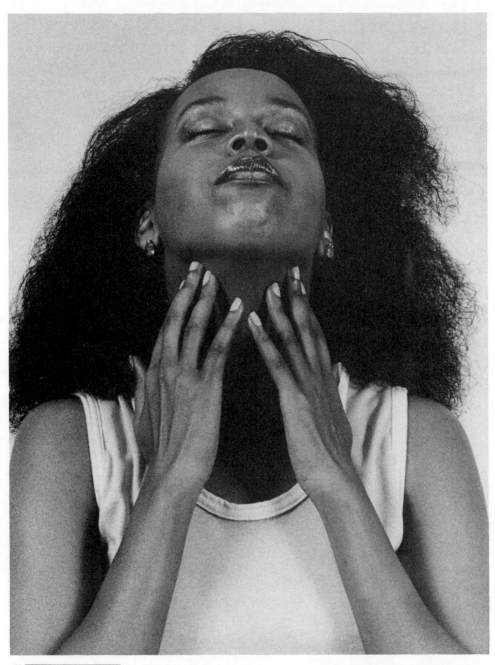

R̲u̲b̲b̲i̲n̲g̲ out the wrinkles in neck and chin. Use long, firm, stroking motions from base of neck up to chin.

154   MASSAGE TECHNIQUES

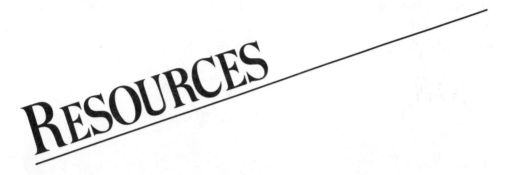

RESOURCES

Prudden, Bonnie. *Pain Erasure the Bonnie Prudden Way*. New York: M. Evans and Company, Inc., 1980.

Hansen, Richard. *Get Well At Home*. Collegedale, Tenn.: College Press, 1980.

Tranquility Tank. 141 Fifth Avenue, 8th Floor, New York, NY 10010; (212-475-5225).

AUNU. Ansonia Station #1206, New York, NY 10023.

Acupressure. Michael Gach, 2533 Shattuck Avenue, Berkeley, CA 94709.

Rubenfeld Synergy. Illana Rubenfeld, 15 Waverly Place, New York, NY 10011 (212-254-5100).

Reflexology. Bill Flocco, 4070 W. Third Street, Los Angeles, CA 90020 (213-389-4424).

Laura Norman, 2 East 37th Street, New York, NY 10016 (212-532-4404).

Sports Massage. Dr. M. K. Hungerford, 120 East 18th Street, Costa Mesa, CA 92627 (714-645-7942).

Polarity. Lewis Harrison, 40 West 72nd Street, New York, NY 10023.

Shiatsu. Deborah Shikora, 205 W. 95th Street, New York, NY 10025.

Swedish Institute, 875 Avenue of the Americas, New York, NY 10001.

Hydrotherapy. Dr. Richard Hanson, Poland Springs, ME (207-998-2894).

Swedish Massage. American Massage and Therapy Association (for list of local therapists or approved schools).

Marilyn Frender (editor of AMTA journal), 200 W. 58th Street, New York, NY 10022.

Susan Stone, 1401 East Lincoln, Royal Oak, MI 48067.

Myotherapy. Institute for Physical Fitness, Stockbridge, MA 01262 (413-298-3066).

Therapeutic Touch. Dr. Delores Kreiger, Division of Nursing, NYU, 50 W. 4th Street, New York, NY 10003.

Esthetic Massage. DBL International, 1990 Broadway, #1206, New York, NY 10023.

Index

(Italic folios indicate illustrations)

Abdomen, 46, 48, 72
    massage, 51, 52, 60, 63, 100
Acupressure, 14, 31–32, 39, 45–
        48, 92
    certification in, 48
    history of, 31–32
    law and, 48
    macroreflexology and, 70
    practitioners of, 48, 91
    schools for, 48
Acupressure (Michael Gach), 155
Acupuncture, 31, 70, 73
Alberta, Angela, 68
Alexander, Frederick Matthias,
        105
Alexander Technique, 102–17
    background, 105–06
    benefits of, 102–05
    careers in, 116
    certification for, 116
    practitioners of, 109, 112, 117
    principles of, 106, 108–09
    schools for, 116
    techniques of, 107, 109, *110–
        11*, 112, *113–15*
Alliance for Massage Thera-
        pists, 43
Alternating baths, 121

American Center for the Alex-
        ander Technique
        (ACAT), 116, 117
American Massage Therapy
        Association (AMTA),
        43, 66, 67, 68, 69, 156
American Massage Therapy In-
        stitute, 17, 30
Amma, 34
Arm, 22, *57*, 72, 98, 126
AUNU Herbal Sauna, 125
AUNU (skin-care products),
        134, 146, 155

Back, 22, *27*, 28, 45–46, 104
    Alexander Technique and,
        104, *111, 113*
    friction (massage) for, *61*
    myotherapy and, 93, *97,* 98,
        100
    petrissage of, 60
    reflexology and, 72
    vibration and, 63
Backaches, 21, 34, *42*, 45–46
Baths
    alternating, 121
    foot, 124
    steam, 120

Beating (massage), 61
Bodo (wooden dowel), 95
Body stretch, 28
Body systems, 10–15, 55
    See also specific systems
Bodywork, 9, 10, 66, 90
    hydrotherapy, 120
    reflexology, 72, 73, 91
    Shiatsu, 31–45
Bowers, Dr. Edwin F., 72
Brackett, Louise, 68
Bun-shin (Shiatsu), 37

Carrington, Walter, 116
Carrington School, 116
Carter, Mildred, 72
Chest, 22, 46, 122, 126
Chiropractors, 66, 91
Chuaka, 14
Circulation, improved, 32, 40,
        49, 55, 60, 63, 71, *83,*
        118, 119, 120, 121, 124,
        126, 130, 137, 140, 142,
        145, 146, 151
Circulatory system, 13, 51, 55
Clapping (massage), 61
Colon
    benefits of massage, 13, 51,

Colon (*cont.*)
    52, 104, 122
    spastic, 13, 93
Colonic irrigation, 122
Compresses, 122–*23, 124,* 146
Conception vessel, 36
Cupping (massage), 61

Dahlgrer, Albert E., 68
Digestive system, 13, 51, 52, 55,
    104, 122
Do-shin (Shiatsu), 37

Ears
    esthetic massage, 147, *152*
    (micro) reflexology, 70, 72,
        73, 74, 75, 76, *81,* 90, 91
Eastern theory, 73–74
Education of the American
    Massage Therapy Asso-
    ciation, 17
Effleurage, 55–*56, 57,* 60, 63,
    65, 121
Elbow
    effleurage for, *57*
    injury, sports, 22
    tennis, 21, 57, 93–94
Enton Hall Clinic, 119
Esthetic massage, 128–54
    background of, 128
    benefits of, 130, 135, 136
    equipment for, 141, 146
    practitioners of, 129
    techniques, 129, 142, *144,*
        146–54
    treatments, 135–37, *138–39,*
        140–41, 142, *143, 153*
Esthetic Massage (DBL Interna-
    tional), 156
Eyes, 22, 24
    esthetic massage for, *149, 153*

Face
    anatomy of, *131*
    esthetic massage for, 128,
        129–30, *147*
    exercise for, 137, *138–39*
    facelift, 140
    myotherapy and, 98
    packs for, 146
    problems, 134–35, 142, 150
    reflexology and, 72
    treatment for, 125, 135–37,
        138–39, 140–41, 142,
        143–53
    vibration and, 63

Facial massage, 140–*43, 147–53*
    equipment, 141
Farmers, Martha, 67
Feet, 22
    Alexander Technique and,
        114
    effleurage for, *57*
    esthetic massage and, 129
    myotherapy and, 95
    petrissage for, 60
    reflexology and, 70, *71,* 72–
        76, *80–84,* 85, *86–87,* 88,
        89, 90–91
Feidenkraus, Moshe, *103*
Fender, Marilyn, 156
Fingers, 22, 93
Fitzgerald, Dr. William H., 72,
    74
Flocco, Bill, *71,* 91, 155
Fomentations (hydrotherapy),
    122
Foot Fixer (Clairol), 88
Footbath, *124*
Fracture, 22, 50, 61, 90
Friction (massage), 60–*61,* 65,
    120

Get Well at Home (Richard Han-
    sen), 119, 120, 155
Governing vessel, 36
Grasp technique, 76–77
Guild Hall, 106

Hacking (massage), 61
Hair, esthetic massage and,
    129, *151*
Hall, Judy E., Ph.D., 68
Hand, 28
    effleurage for, *57*
    esthetic massage and, 129
    myotherapy and, 95
    petrissage for, 60
    (micro) reflexology and, 70,
        72, 73, 74, 76, *77–80,* 90,
        91
Hansen, Richard A., M.D., 119,
    120
Hara (Shiatsu), 38–41
Harrison, Lewis, 155
Head, 22, 24
    headaches, 21, 47, 63, 64, 93,
        121
    myotherapy and, 98
    vibration and, 63
Head roll, 98
Heat packs, 65

Heel lift, 100
Hippocrates, 10
"Hook and Pull" technique,
    76–77
Hospital Yerba Buena, 119
Hot tubs, 125
Hungerford, Marquetta K.,
    Ph.D., 17, 30, 155
Hydrotherapy, 24, 54, 95, 118–
    27, 128, 130, 146
    background, 119
    baths, 120–21
    benefits of, 118–19, 120–22,
        124
    careers in, 127
    certification, 127
    clinics, 119
    equipment for, 118, 120, 124,
        125, 126, 146
    principles of, 120
    schools, 126–27
    techniques, 120–26
    therapists, 121, 127
Hydrotherapy, 156

"Inchworm" technique, 76, *80*
Ingham, Eunice, 72
Institute for Physical Fitness
    and Myotherapy, 94,
    101, 156
International Myotherapy Asso-
    ciation, 101

Jitsu (Shiatsu), 38–39, 40
Joints, 20, 21, 23, 61, 64, 106
    disorders, 48, 104
    friction (massage), 60
    mobility, 13, 50, 55

Kellogg, John Harvey, 119
Kenbiki (Shiatsu), 40
Ki, 14, 36
Kidneys, 14, 52, 135
Kinesthetic sense, 108, 112
Kneading. *See* Muscles, knead-
    ing; Petrissage.
Knee, 21, 24
    exercises, 98, 100
    hydrotherapy, 122
    injury, sports, 22, 24
    protective gear, 24
    stretch, *27*
    technique, massage, 64
Kreiger, Dr. Delores, 156
Kyo (Shiatsu), 38, 39

Laura Norman & Associates, 91

Laws, massage, 41, 66–69
Legs
  cramps, preventing, *25*
  effleurage and, *56*
  esthetic massage and, 129
  exercise for, 24, *26, 27–28, 29,
    42,* 99, 126
  injury, sports, 22
  myotherapy and, *96, 97*
  reflexology and, 72
  vibration and, 63
Lemocks, Bill, 67
Licensing. *See* Massage, laws;
    *specific techniques, certifica-
    tion*
Ling, Peter Hendrik, 53
Lungs, 52, 63
Lymphatic system, 55, 118

McClanaghan, Robert W., 69
McDonald, Patrick, 116
McDonald School, 116
Macroreflexology, 70
Massage, 11, 54, 55, 64, 65, 66,
    72
  avoid, 17, 51, 90
  baby, 100, 109
  benefits, 10, 13, 50, 52, 53
  equipment, 64–65, 88, 95,
    112, 118, 120, 121, 124,
    125, 126, 141, 146
  laws, 41, 48, 66–69, 76, 91
  paralysis, 16, 53, 61
  systems, 14
  See also specific techniques
Masunaga, Shizuto, 34
Matrix holdouts, 98
Melander, Captain Theodore,
    66
Meridians, energy, 31, 32, 34,
    35, 36, 37, 38, 39, 40, 42,
    45, 73–74
Microreflexology, 70
Mon-shin (Shiatsu), 38
Moss, Jason, 80
Mount Akagi Institute, 119
Muscle squeeze, *83*
Muscles
  abdominal, 27, 29, 46
  Alexander Technique and,
    104
  beauty, maintaining, 140
  benefits of massage to, 13,
    50–51, 60
  esthetic massage and, 130
  friction (massage) to, 60, 61

hydrotherapy and, 118
kneading and, 18, *19, 23*
reeducation of, 48
reflexology and, 73, 76
short, 60, 108
strengthening, 27–28, 100,
    127
tapotement (massage) and,
    63
tears to, 21, 22, 26
Muscular system, 11, *12,* 13, 49,
    55, 104
Myotherapy, 73, 92–101
  background, 93–94
  benefits of, 92–93
  careers in, 101
  certification for, 98, 100, 101
  equipment for, 95
  Institute for, 94, 101
  menstrual troubles and, 93,
    96, 104
  practitioners of, 98, 100, 101
  principles of, 94–95
  schools for, 101
  self-help and, 98, *99,* 100
  techniques, 95, *96–97,* 99
Myotherapy (Institute for Physi-
    cal Fitness), 156
Myotherapy: Pain-free Living
    (video by Bonnie Prud-
    den), 94

Namikoshi, Tokujiro, 34
Neck, *25,* 46, *111*
  Alexander Technique and,
    110, 111, 114
  esthetic massage and, 146
  injury, sports, 22
  myotherapy and, 93
  reflexology and, 72
  Shiatsu and, 34, *43*
  vibration and, 63, *64*
Nerves, 50, 60, 63, 70, 73
Nervous system, 13, 52, 53, 73,
    94, 95, 118
New College of Speech and
    Drama, 106
Nogier, Dr., 72
Norman, Laura, 155

Ohashiatsu (Shiatsu), 34
Osteopathy, 14

*Pain Erasure the Bonnie Prudden
    Way* (Bonnie Prudden),
    94, 155

Palming (Shiatsu), 40
Petrissage, 58–59, 60, 63, 121
Polarity, 14, 73, 155
Polarity (Lewis Harrison), 155
Posture, 27
  Alexander Technique and,
    104, *107, 110*
  esthetic massage and, 136
  poor, results of, 46, 94
Practitioner/Therapist. *See spe-
    cific techniques*
President's Council on Physical
    Fitness and Sports, 94
Pressure points, 31, *44, 45,* 92,
    98, 132
Prudden, Bonnie, 92, 93, 94, 98,
    100

Range of motion, 18, *20,* 21, 40,
    55
Reflex points, *77–87,* 89
Reflexology, 70–91, 155
  background, 72
  careers in, 90–91
  cautions against, 76, 90
  certification for, 90
  equipment for, 88
  imbalance and, 72, 73–74, *75*
  license, 76
  microreflexology and, 70
  philosophy of, 72–74
  practitioner of, 76, 91
  reflex points and, *77–87*
  schools for, 90–91
  self-applied, *89,* 90
  systems of, 73, 74, *75,* 76
  techniques, 76, *77, 78–87,* 88,
    90
Reflexology (Bill Flocco), 155
Reflexology Workshop, 80, 91
Respiratory system, 13, 14, 55
Riley, Dr. Joseph, 72
Rolfing, 14
Royal Academy of Dramatic
    Art, 106
Royal College of Music, 106
Royal Institute of Gymnastics,
    53
Rubenfeld, Illana, *103,* 155
Rubenfeld Synergy (Illana Ruben-
    feld), 155

Saunas, 146
Scalp, 72, *151*
Schools. *See specific techniques*
Seat lift, 100

Self-exercise, 27, 28
Self-massage, 28, *29*, 34, 65, 89,
90, 95, 98, *99*, 100, 126,
129, 141, 142, *152–54*
Serizawa, Katsusuke, 34
Setsu-shin (Shiatsu), 38
Shiatsu, 31–45, 155
benefits of, 32, 34
careers in, 41–43
certification, 41, 43
history, 34
imbalances and, 32, 35, 37,
39, 41
licensing for, 41
practitioners of, 31–32, 41,
43, 91
principles of, 35–39
schools for, 41, 43
self-techniques, *47*
techniques, 40–41, *47*
Shiatsu, 155
Shoulders, 21, *25*, 46
Alexander Technique and,
114
esthetic massage and, 150
injury, sports, 22
muscle kneading for, *23*
protective gear for, 24
Shiatsu and, *43*
vibration and, *64*
Sit-ups, 27
Sitz bath, 120
Skeletal system, 10, *11*, 55
Skin, 22, 65
anatomy, *133*
benefits of massage, 50, 54–
55
esthetic massage, 129, 140,
142, *151*
facts, basic, 132–34
hydrotherapy, 125
products for care of, 134
reflexology, 70
Smith, Peggy G., 69
Society for Teachers of the
Alexander Technique
(STAT), 116
Spasms, 11, 16, 46, 92, 94, 95,
98, 121

Spine, *11*, 46, 48, 73, 115
Alexander Technique and,
104, 106, *111, 113*
vibration and, 63
Sports massage, 16–30, 64, 66–
67, 94, 155
background, 17
benefits of, 16–17, 21, 22, *24,
27*
careers in, 30
certification, 30
principles and philosophy of,
17–18
schools, 30
techniques, 18–30
therapists, 30
Sports Massage (Dr. M. K. Hungerford), 155
Sprains, 21, 22, 46, 61
Steam baths, 120
Steam inhalation, 124
Steam rooms, 146
Stockbridge Institute, 93
Stomach, 22, 29, *84*
Stress, 9, 18, 32, 36, 51, 53, 67,
71, 104
Stretching, *24, 25, 26, 27*, 28, *42,
47*
Swedish Institute, 66, 155
Swedish massage, 49–69
background, 51–54, 64
benefits of, 49–53, 55, 61, 63,
66
careers, 65–67
certification. *See* Swedish
massage, laws.
injuries, aided by, 50, 51
laws for, 66–69
principles of, 54–55
schools, 65, 66, 156
techniques, 55–65, 66, 120–
21
therapists, 64, 65, 66, 67
Swimming (hydrotherapy), 126

Tanks, flotation/isolation, 125–
26
Taping, 23, 24
Tapotement, 61, *62*, 63, 121

Tapping, 61
Tension, 10, 11, 28, 29, 48
Alexander Technique and,
102, 106, 112, 113
effleurage and, *56–57*
esthetic massage and, 135,
136, 140, 141, 142, 150
hydrotherapy and, 120, 125–
26
myotherapy and, 96
petrissage and, 121
reflexology and, *83*
Shiatsu and, 31–45
Swedish massage and, 65
tapotement and, 63
Therapeutic Touch (Dr. Delores
Kreiger), 156
Therapist/Practitioner. *See spe-
cific techniques*
"Thumb walk," 76, *80*
Thumbing (Shiatsu), 40
Tivey, Dr. Desmond R., 93
Tranquility Tank, 155
Travell, Janet, M.D., 93
Trigger point injection therapy,
93
Trigger points, 92, 93, 94, 95,
96, 97, 98
Tsubos (Shiatsu), 35, 38

Urinary system, 14

V-sit, 27
Vaporizer, 125
Vibration (massage), 63, *64*,
121
Visualization, beauty, 141–42

Water-Pik, 121
Western theory, 73
Whirlpools, 125, 146
White, Dr. George Starr, 72
Wildwood Sanitarium and Hos-
pital, 127
Wrist, 22, 28, 72, 122

Zone theory, 73, 74
Zone therapy, 70, 72, 73, 74
Zones, 74, *75*, 76